# Life in Rewind

# LIFE IN REWIND

The Story of a Young Courageous Man

Who Persevered Over OCD and the Harvard

Doctor Who Broke All the Rules to Help Him

◀◀

TERRY WEIBLE MURPHY

WITH Edward E. Zine AND Michael A. Jenike, M.D.

*wm*

WILLIAM MORROW

*An Imprint of* HarperCollins*Publishers*

FIRST EDITION

*Designed by Richard Oriolo*

Library of Congress Cataloging-in-Publication Data has been
applied for.

ISBN 978-0-06-156153-5

09 10 11 12 13 OV/RRD 10 9 8 7 6 5 4 3 2 1

FOR PATRICK—

*in whose extraordinary wisdom, grace, and love*

*I find my greatest strength*

# CONTENTS

## ACKNOWLEDGMENTS

In February of 1998, I sat in a quiet restaurant in Clayton, Missouri, across from a man I barely knew, but would never forget, and announced that one day I would write a book. It was an improbable dream, and I'm still not sure whether I was selling the idea to him, or to myself, but clearly the seed took root. Exactly ten years later, in February of 2008, I delivered the manuscript for this book to my publisher at HarperCollins.

The journey from that moment to this began with a belief system that was instilled in me by my mother, Carol, who was a gifted "believer" in her children. She was a voracious reader—and that included every little poem and story that I scribbled for her in crayon, pencil, or ink, or plunked into type. She just *knew* I was a writer, and that one day everyone else would know, too. She is, no doubt, celebrating with my father, cheek to cheek, dancing in the great beyond.

At the heart of every word I've written in this book is my son, Patrick. From the moment of his birth, he has been my greatest teacher, informing my understanding and deep appreciation of God, courage, truth, love, and the incongruity found in the power and fragility of life. He was a child with special needs who grew into a man of many special gifts. He is my hero, and the world is a better place because he is alive and well.

Lori, Jeff, Mark, Ron, and Rick—from the youngest to the oldest—there has never been a way to escape their love and support at every turn of my life, even at times when I tried. I have been blessed to grow up in this large, loving Weible family, because I always knew that whenever I fell, there would be someone to pick me up, and love me just the same.

Jim Murphy—if I've not said it enough in the span of our lifetime of knowing one another, thank you for encouraging me to go back to college, for being a great father, and for sharing your wonderful parents, Anna and Jim, whom I still love as my own.

I thank my friend Laura Muench who inspired me to believe I could be more than one cranky old man's secretary (not that there's anything wrong with being a secretary, there's not; it was the cranky old man who was the problem). Nunzio Edward—I thank you for being a truly wonderful friend whose love and support helped keep me sane, relatively speaking.

My agent and friend Babette Perry paid attention for all the years I threw out one idea after another; I don't know why, since most of them fell flat, but she did. And it is because she listened, and believed in the possibility of this story, that it has come to life. She is a woman with an extraordinary heart and mind, and she manages to navigate the world of entertainment with an incomparable integrity and grace.

Lisa Sharkey had been on the job at HarperCollins for only a couple of weeks when I first got the call that she was interested in *Life in Rewind*. She knew Dr. Michael Jenike from her days as a television producer, and there is no one in whose hands this book would be better served than Lisa's. She has been a great, intuitive guide throughout this process, and she gifted me with the perfect editor in Adam Korn. I watched as Adam fell in love with the story of Dr. Michael Jenike and Ed Zine . . . it was a literary dance through which he led me safely to an intelligent compilation of words, sentences, and chapters that tell the story in the most compelling way possible. I thank him for his enormous patience and creativity.

To Duff—I thank you for helping pick me up off the floor when I was thoroughly exhausted from writing this book.

And last, but certainly not least, to Michael Jenike, a man with whom I can always, most respectfully, agree to disagree, and still hopelessly admire. And Ed—your genius is unfathomable, and I thank you for the long hours in which you honored and entrusted me with your beautiful story.

## MICHAEL A. JENIKE, M.D.

⏪

IT HAS BEEN MANY YEARS since I first met Ed Zine at his house on Cape Cod. He suffered from a most severe form of an illness that I had studied and treated for more than three decades— obsessive compulsive disorder, or OCD. Ed was as ill as any patient I had ever met. His story, his suffering, and his recovery reveal an inspiring young man who has touched my life in a way I had never expected. I met Terry Murphy while I was consulting for a charitable foundation in New York City. I saw some of the brilliant videos and writing that she had done for the foundation, and remember one of the secretaries being reduced to tears when she viewed one of Terry's videos about the foundation's director. She has a knack for poignantly capturing the most pristine essence of a person.

Ed had spoken many times about having someone write his story as an inspiration to other severely ill OCD patients who had given up hope. If he could get better, anyone could. I told Terry about Ed, and she became enthused and offered to work with Ed to write his story. During the course of writing and working with Ed on his story, she asked me why I became so involved with Ed. She pried into my own motivation and reasons why I would be willing to do things differently from most physicians. I had known from my early years that I was willing to do unusual things to help patients. I had even been criticized during my training for making house calls—"Dr. Jenike gets overinvolved with his patients" wrote one supervisor when commenting on my visits to housebound patients. Because I had been in the military for five years and was older, these comments had absolutely no bearing on how I was going to practice medicine, and to this day I make house calls.

However, Terry astutely detected parallels between my life and traumas and Ed's life. Her teasing apart these issues has allowed me to understand my own motivations in light of my past life. This book reveals more about me than I would like, but I felt I had to step up to the plate and be as brave as Ed, for the benefit of patients who suffer from this horrible illness, as well as for the dedicated physicians who treat them.

I suppose the bottom line is that we all have our traumas, histories, motivations, and accomplishments. If this story touches and motivates you like it has touched Ed and me, then Terry will have accomplished more than I ever expected.

# Life in Rewind

# CHAPTER I

# Leave No Man Behind

THE PIECE OF LINT HAS been missing for nearly a week. Before its sudden disappearance, it lay coupled with the wilted brown leaf on the basement floor near the back door. Its absence is devastating.

Finally, at the end of a long, tedious search, the particle of fluff is discovered, attached to the delicate hind leg of a cricket that has found its way indoors during the rainy season. The exorcism of lint is done with great care, leaving the cricket unharmed. But reconstructing the comfortable universe where the piece of lint once existed with the brittle leaf takes many anguish-filled hours to complete.

Michael Jenike knows nothing of this as he dribbles the bas-

ketball and pushes through the sweaty bodies of the other players barreling toward him, their rubber soles squeaking against
the gym floor as he defends his turf. The tired, but enthusiastic
grunts of grown men meld with the pounding rhythm of the ball
slamming against their hands, and briefly, they are able to recapture the carefree satisfaction that belonged to them on the
basketball courts of their youth.

After the game, adrenaline still pumping, Michael drops
his gym bag into the back of his new BMW-Z3, slides his six-
feet, two-inch frame behind the wheel, cranks up some country
music, and pushes the speed limit down Route 3 toward Cape
Cod where, on this spring day in 1996, his life will intersect with
a seemingly impenetrable boundary, and he will be forced to confront pieces of his own painful past.

At the same time, the young man who meticulously extracted
the piece of lint from the leg of the cricket sits in the basement
of a modest raised-ranch house, in a wooded, middle-class neighborhood on the coast of Cape Cod, Massachusetts. He can't get
out, and he refuses to let anyone in. The seasons have changed,
schoolchildren who board the bus outside his door have been pro-
moted from one grade to the next, and each day, strangers pass
by without giving a moment's thought to what's happening behind
the closed door at the bottom of the thirteen steps on the side of
the quiet house.

Isolated from friends who think he's away at college, he sits on
the end of his bed, rocking back and forth, helplessly performing
repetitive rituals of forward and backward counting, all multiples
of even numbers that stretch well into the tens of thousands. The
cable television guide that rolls on the screen in front of him is
his only gauge for the time that passes, as he sits with his hands

outstretched from his body, fingers spread, locked into position like the claws of an eagle, while his mind rages with the repetitive pounding of a terrible equation that will not let him go.

*Time equals Progression, Progression equals Death.* This is the mantra that keeps twenty-four-year-old Ed Zine living on the end of a mental tether with invisible strands attached to every muscle, thought, and spoken word. This tether is his safety net, rewinding and erasing every action that would otherwise propel him forward in time. When the rewind is complete, he is given momentary relief from the anxiety of the equation with which he is so preoccupied.

Ed's obsession is logic gone completely awry. Although it's true that the time line of our lives follows this sequence of *Time equals Progression, Progression equals Death,* few of us ever scrutinize each moment and each movement as a path to our certain end. Surely, such torture would drive us mad. For Ed, who suffers from severe obsessive-compulsive disorder, the perpetual rewinding is a ritual; more aptly, a series of rituals within rituals, which temporarily relieves the madness his intrusive thoughts create. Assaulted by this logical, but paralyzing notion, his illogical mind creates a battle that rages within him every second of every day.

Early in the day, Ed began moving from the end of his bed toward the basement door in anticipation of Michael Jenike's arrival. It is a daunting task that takes him nearly seven hours to complete, and all the while he wonders if this is the one person who will release him from this personal hell.

Dr. Michael Jenike is a professor of psychiatry at Harvard Medical School and one of the world's leading experts in the research and treatment of obsessive-compulsive disorder. He describes OCD as a disorder of "pure suffering," and he brings to its treatment not only an extraordinary scientific mind, but also a profound depth of compassion for his patients. The message from his secretary is simple: a young man is stuck in his basement and needs help. She knows that Michael's already busy schedule doesn't really allow him to take a full day to see a new patient, but she also knows that nothing she says will stop him from going. Someone is trapped, and that's really all Michael needs to know as he pushes his own life clock forward, driving almost three hours to meet his new patient.

After a brief introduction to the Zine family—who are gathered on the front lawn to greet him, amazed that he has come all this way to respond to their call for help—Michael walks slowly up the driveway along the washed-out gray privacy fence as tentatively as he might test the ice of a newly frozen pond. He cannot see his new patient standing inside the basement at the bottom of the steps, but he does hear the instructions being issued through a small six-inch opening in the door. Ed will not allow Michael into the basement, nor will he allow him to walk into the twenty-foot perimeter outside the basement door, which he describes as his "OCD Holy Ground." Before Michael can even breech that perimeter, he is asked to stop.

Michael's goal this day is to simply start by building an alliance with Ed. "A lot of times, when people are stuck, they have all kinds of rituals that they're afraid you're going to interfere with," he says, "so you have to find out what world they're living in, and join it for a while. I wanted to be cautious, listen to what his rules were, and try not to violate them."

If Michael moves too quickly, or changes the placement of even the smallest leaf in Ed's OCD Holy Ground, there is little hope for an alliance because it will have upended Ed's entire sacred universe, setting in motion a series of physical and mental rituals to rewind and secure the placement of the leaf to its original state, just as he did with the lint that the cricket moved. "The lint and the leaf gave me solace," Ed recalls. "Keeping my world exactly as it was kept that good feeling in place. I felt like, right there, everything was comfortable, and nothing bad was going to happen to anybody. When the lint moved, I lost control of time and events."

Clearly, human contact of any kind is excruciatingly painful for Ed. "It changed everything in my world, and it was physically painful to me," says Ed. "I couldn't bear to have anything around me touched or moved." This was the prelude to Ed's isolation, his inability to allow anyone near him who might brush up against him or move the possessions that had become the placekeepers of happy moments in time.

But almost immediately, Ed senses in Michael a level of care and respect for his pain that he's not felt from other medical professionals he's encountered. "Dr. Jenike had the presence of mind not to invade the grounds which were, to me, so unstained. At the same time, though, I had to let him know what the parameters were. I couldn't let him inside. I had to tell him, 'I don't feel comfortable, and you have to stay there.'"

Michael takes a seat on the ground and gently begins to build on that tiny fraction of trust. Even from this distance, talking through a closed door, he is able to evaluate the depth of Ed's disorder without ever setting eyes on him. Ed exhibits classic signs of severe OCD—intrusive thoughts, repetitive counting and checking, contamination issues, and hoarding. But Michael discovers another alarming distinction in the way OCD holds his new patient captive. Ed Zine believes through his strict regimen of rituals—which is essentially organized chaos—he can stop the progression of time.

Ed's OCD mind has convinced him that by reversing every action, he can alter the equation of *Time equals Progression, Progression equals Death*. He figures that if he can protect his time and space by reversing the actions, and if he can, in his own mind, erase events, as if they had never happened, he will be able to prevent time from moving forward and all those people he loves will remain young, healthy, and . . . alive. It is never about protecting himself from death, it is always about others.

The madness of OCD is that while the irrational mind is operating, its victim is able to observe and recognize this behavior. It is a neurologically based anxiety disorder with symptoms that often look "crazy" to outside observers, but the sufferer isn't crazy at all. Individuals who suffer with OCD know that their illogical behavior has no logical basis, and knowing this increases their suffering all the more, because without treatment they are unable to stop it.

Imagine Ed as a child standing on the shore watching the other kids swim and play without a care in the world. He wants nothing more than to jump in and splash around in the "normal" waters that beckon him from just a few feet away, but his swim trunks are covered by layers of winter clothing. He knows it makes absolutely no sense that he's wearing winter clothing on a hot summer day, but he is incapable of shedding his woolen wear to get down to the layers of cotton clothing that make sense for summer and swimming.

Multiple layers of simultaneous thought are occurring at lightning speed in the narrow partition between Ed's logical and illogical minds as he monitors his physical and mental activity. During the seven-hour journey from his bed to the door leading outside where Michael now sits trying to get to know him, Ed's brain continuously scans his physical environment for changes, information downloaded from television, and dialogue with members of his family who drop off food outside the basement door, checking and rechecking his mechanisms for holding time in its place hundreds and thousands of times. The fifteen-foot trip across the room is an excruciating testament to this process:

*Right foot forward, left foot, right foot forward, left . . . a truck passes by . . . freeze. Left foot still in air, hold perfectly still for one and a half hours and wait for another truck to pass by that sounds exactly the same. With conditions now perfect, reverse process, and go backward to starting place to do it all over from beginning. Left foot down, step backward in same exact spot, now right foot backward, left . . . no. Stop. The fingers of your right hand touched. Freeze. Count in multiples of even numbers all the way to 16,384, and back, touching and untouching your fingers dozens of times to fix mistake. Move your feet into exact position they were in when your fingers touched, then reverse all moves back to spot where truck passed by. Wait. Keep fingers locked so they don't touch. Freeze. Wait fifteen more minutes until another truck passes by. Start again. Right, left, right, left. Was big toe on right foot pointed in exact position for second step as it was for first? No. Go backward. Freeze. Wait. Does everything feel right? Okay, start again. A dog barks. Freeze. Wait until dog barks, again. . . .*

In much the same way one describes an out-of-body experience, Ed has watched himself descend into this extraordinary underground life in his father's basement where his mind holds him hostage.

IT'S POSSIBLE THAT ONE OF the most effective tools in Michael Jenike's medical kit is his disarming sense of humor. Still, he is surprised to find that Ed, as sick as he is, responds, albeit weakly, to Michael's self-effacing jokes, and he has his own sense of humor, too. After hours of talking through the basement door, Ed begins to feel slightly more comfortable—not comfortable enough to let the doctor into the basement, but comfortable enough to consider meeting him face-to-face in the upper level of the house. Michael is given instructions to follow as he comes around the front of the house through the main door, turning the handle back and forth repeatedly, ending on an even number, because odd numbers are bad, and opening and closing the door an even number of times, too, before coming inside. Michael must wait for a considerable period of time as Ed struggles up the few wooden steps, stopping and starting, going forward and backward, as he counts in multiples of even numbers to 16,384. Ed is ashamed of the way he looks, and agreeing to come upstairs creates added layers of anxiety that result in more counting, and more repeating of his steps.

Just four years earlier, Ed was a tall, good-looking athlete, who was determined to try out as a walk-on for the Clemson University football team. It was a long shot of a dream for the lanky kid with an undistinguished high school playing career, but he had a powerful throwing arm and had managed to get the attention of one of the team's coaches. He took classes at the local community college and worked out every night at the gym to build his strength and develop his body, but the version of Ed Zine who emerges from the basement is someone completely different—at least in appearance

Michael tries to catch his breath. The stench of body waste and rot come back to him from another place and time. Flashbacks and nausea consume him. From the stairwell below, a rancid breeze blows through the air, emanating from piles of human feces stored in Ziploc bags, meshed with the odor of dozens of Gatorade bottles overflowing with ripe urine. But that is only part of the sickening smell. The frail, hunched-over shadow walking up the stairs, forward and backward, has not showered, shaved, or brushed his teeth in nearly a year. Ed's eyes are squinted shut from the sudden exposure to bright light, and his long, curly hair is matted against his crusted scalp, sticking out in every direction. Pale and undernourished, he drowns in his dirty white T-shirt and gray sweatpants, neither of which he's changed for months.

Fighting the urge to vomit, Michael tries to reconcile the sight and smell of this desperately ill young man covered in bedsores, who seems more akin to a wild, injured animal emerging from its den than the gentle, respectful young man he's spent the last few hours getting to know. Obsessive-compulsive disorder has completely stripped Ed of his dignity and of the basic ability to cleanse his body and put on clean clothes.

Ed makes his way to the family room, and for brief periods during this conversation, he suddenly disengages and goes into some kind of trance, mouthing words silently to himself. The interruptions are brought on by his need to repeat his spoken words backward several times, until he meets a perfect rewind and achieves the final even number of repetitions. Incredibly, Ed Zine has taught himself to read and speak backward. He has mastered perfect English, in reverse. His fluency is extraordinary. He can read this sentence as quickly backward as he can forward.

*.drawrof nac eh sa drawkcab ylkciuq sa ecnetnes siht daer nac eH*

The obsession to stop the progression of time and the thousands upon thousands of resulting rituals have turned Ed's mind into a photographic and audiological masterpiece trained on the relentless pursuit of perfection.

Ed and Michael are engaged in a two-way psychological assessment. While Ed is continuing his silent rituals, he is also actively analyzing Michael. He is very wary of anyone new. Recently, he suffered what he feels was a betrayal by his family who had assumed, incorrectly (and quite ironically), that he was a suicide risk and had him committed to the local psychiatric hospital. As much as he wants help to get his life back, he does not want someone who is going to *demand* his trust; he needs someone he can *believe in*. According to Ed, there's a critical distinction. "Believing in somebody means that they give *you* the ability and have the faith that *you* can make your decisions along the way. When we got upstairs and really talked, it hit me, 'BOOM,' this is someone I can really believe in."

In the living room that day, the conversation between doctor and patient did not focus on OCD—there was no need, Ed already knew his diagnosis. Instead, it was an afternoon of relationship building, as Ed shared with Michael the details of his solitary life. He sprinkles the conversation with questions to his new doctor. Is he married? Does he have children? Ed talks about his recent hospitalization, and honor—one of his favorite subjects—and he discovers that Michael is a war veteran, a pilot who served in the air force in Vietnam. In all of this, there is nothing about Michael's presence that says, "I'm the doctor, you're the patient."

But he is the doctor, and with that he has brought all the years of his considerable experience to bear in that meeting, and he has never seen anyone with OCD this severe. "Ed was very sick, and really stuck. He was so trapped in circular thinking, there was no angle that could be used to help him." But on this first day, Michael hasn't come to see Ed with a big game plan in mind; he is there to make an assessment, form an alliance, and determine whether Ed is able to come to the Obsessive Compulsive Disorder Institute at McLean Hospital for residential treatment. But it is clear that such a move is not possible.

At the end of the day, Michael knows that although Ed wants to get well, "he wasn't going to move for anybody else's ideas and thoughts other than his own. I hoped if we got to know one another better, and tried some medicine and behavioral therapy, we could get him out of there."

If anyone can help Ed, it is Michael. He has the best skill and experience that medicine has to offer, but over the course of the next year, he will discover there are no easy answers. He will watch helplessly as his young patient spirals deeper and deeper into his own mind, haunted by that echoing equation, *Time equals Progression, Progression equals Death,* and the ever-increasing rituals OCD demands of him. Ed will eventually stop wearing clothes altogether and spend most of his time sitting undressed on the end of his bed watching television, rewinding movies backward and forward, while the unwashed sheets oxidize to a shimmering green slime from the filth of body oils and droppings of food. Helping Ed will prove Michael's biggest challenge in twenty years of treating some of the most extreme documented cases of OCD.

**IN SPITE OF WHAT WOULD** become his growing belief that Ed might never get better, and would most likely spend the rest of his life living in the basement of his father's home, Michael would continue his visits, driving the distance between Boston and Cape Cod over and over because he knew that no one else would, and he understood his presence mattered in the life of a human being who was suffering inconceivable anguish. He recognized all of the deep, dark feelings that can trap a human mind, for *Captain* Michael Jenike, an honored war hero and recipient of the Distinguished Flying Cross, had also known such depths of despair.

Michael would find himself lost in the hopelessness of Ed's situation. At the end of each visit, he would drive a short distance down the road, pull his car off to the side, turn on the flashers, and cry. It would be a long time before he would realize that deep within him, he possessed everything he needed to lead his patient to a place where the healing process could begin.

# CHAPTER 2

# The Day Life Stopped

◀◀

IN THE PICTURE-PERFECT, WHITE-SHUTTERED two-story with
its welcoming front porch, nestled among tall trees, with delicate
lilac bushes etched against its windows, Rita Zine had created a
gentle, loving environment for her children. It was a place where
Ed could walk into the sunshine on a glorious New England day
and never have to think about stopping time, because *here* time
had no special meaning. He didn't need to worry about things being touched, or moved, because every*one* was safe, and every*thing*
was in its proper place.

And though life inside the Zine household was far from perfect, it *felt* perfect to Ed because his mother made it so. She sang
to him and cooked for him while he sat at the kitchen counter

watching his favorite cartoons on TV. He was her baby boy, and at a time when she was faced with the challenges of an older son who struggled with negative outside influences, she served up an endless stream of affection and support for her youngest, telling Ed that one day, he would do something really important with his life. She snuggled with him while they watched movies together, carried cookies and ice-cold pitchers of lemonade out to the backyard while he played Wiffle ball or swam in the pool. She invited neighborhood children like Rudy Harris, who would later play football for the NFL, to have sandwiches with them after school. Rita was ubiquitous in Ed's happiest memories, and when she would pass away, the tapestry of his life would change *dramatically,* as he would be cared for by his less nurturing, seemingly antithetical father.

Bob Zine was the dark, handsome, volatile son of a Lebanese-born prizefighter-turned-bookie from South Boston who, at age sixteen, forged his mother's signature, lied about his age, and went off to fight for the Marines in World War II. During his induction, as a drill sergeant yelled, "I am your mother and your father, now, son," he was frightened and homesick. Having second thoughts about what he'd done, he called his father to bail him out. "Take it like a man," Bob was told. Whatever gentleness there was inside of him was suppressed that day. His wartime experience would later inform his decisions as a father, and the regimented way he ran his family and home.

After surviving World War II in the Marshall Islands, and serving another term of service in the Korean War, Bob returned home to South Boston where he met, and fell in love with, Rita Grace Nice, a petite blond beauty with a poodle-cut hairdo. Her name perfectly matched her quiet demeanor and style. She was "the prettiest girl in the neighborhood," remembers Bob, "and I fell in love with her the minute I laid eyes on her." The early years of their marriage were lean but loving, as Bob worked long hours as a plumber to support his burgeoning family. Eventually, though, he became a master builder and came to own his own business, enabling his family to move into Boston's suburbs to live "the good life."

Ed remembers his mother's scent. She always smelled "shampoo fresh," mingled at times with smoke from the cigarettes she dangled between her fingers as she sat at the kitchen table playing dominoes and Yahtzee. She was the center of Ed's universe, with television coming in a distant, though *not insignificant,* second.

To this day, Ed can recall the day and time when his favorite shows from the seventies and eighties aired. He never missed programs like *The Incredible Hulk, The Greatest American Hero,* and *Magnum P.I.,* and he developed a passion for the ones that had veritable heroes in the leading role. A quiet, sensitive child, he connected emotionally with their power and honor, and he used the story lines of good and evil to begin developing his own simplistic code of ethics. In one episode of *The Incredible Hulk,* Hulk impersonator Lou Ferrigno stops a man from using physical force against his son, and despite the fact that Ed's father, like so many men of his generation, frequently employed physical discipline to rear his kids, Ed instantly recognized that dads are *not* supposed to hit their children. "In that moment, I realized that it wasn't something that was inherited or predestined," recalls Ed, "and I decided right then and there, I didn't have to be that way. I was never going to hit my children when I grew up."

But it would be a fallacy to paint Bob Zine as chronically abusive. Ed and his father were actually quite close, and they shared many special times during his childhood. On weekends, when his dad was at his most relaxed, away from the stresses of work, Ed would crawl up on the sofa next to him in his pajamas and, together, they would watch the Sunday Night Movie of the Week, movies like *The Dirty Dozen, The Big Red One,* and the *James Bond* movies. Having a father who was an ex-marine and, in Ed's eyes, a real-life hero only served to make the experience more powerful for Ed, allowing him to connect to his father in an emotional and loving way.

But television also became a necessary audio distraction for Ed. Before VCRs were a regular part of the American household, he would take his audiotape player, hold it up close to the television, and record the sound while he watched the show. When the program was over, he would go to his room and play the sound over and over again, rewinding it to his favorite moments, blocking out the arguments his parents would be having in the other room. "I used to see my mom and dad fight, which was very hard, but I chose to look past a lot of it," recalls Ed.

Bob and Rita Zine fought constantly about their oldest son and issues of discipline. Adding to the stress, around this same time, the formerly petite beauty had nearly doubled in size, making her a target for her husband's explosive and often cruel verbal lashings. Unaware that the reason for her weight gain was ovarian cancer, Bob made little secret of the fact that he was planning to leave his wife.

In fact, no one, not even Rita, knew she was sick. Although Ed compares his mother's size and immobility during this time to the profoundly large mother in the movie *What's Eating Gilbert Grape,* he doesn't ever remember being embarrassed by her size, only concerned when she could no longer climb the steps to her bedroom. His older sister Tami recalls, painfully, a comment that her boyfriend made at the time when she told him her dad was going to leave her mom: "If my wife was that big, I would leave her, too."

Ed's last great memory of his mother was a trip to a movie theater in May 1980 when *The Empire Strikes Back* came out. It was a special experience that marked the beginning of his *Star Wars* passion. Shortly after, Rita surprised Ed with a set of *Empire Strikes Back* sheets for his bed and a Darth Vader costume for him to wear at Halloween. Whenever he and his friend Rudy got together to play *Star Wars,* he would put on the full costume and swing his light saber, while his mother joined in the fun with her best imitation . . . "Ahhhhhh, Luke, I am your father!"

But Ed's happier memories are interrupted by later conversations overheard in the kitchen and hallways as he passed by, hushed conversations between his older sisters and aunts when the diagnosis finally came. No one ever said, "Mom has cancer," but Ed knew something was wrong, even if he didn't know exactly what it was. Relatives seemed to always be making an effort to get he and his sister Deena out of the house to do as much "fun stuff" as possible. But for a happy, intuitive young boy to suddenly be pushed away from his mother, watching as she spent more and more of her time in bed, there was little fun in leaving the comfort of his home.

These were the days when *Star Wars* fun and pitchers of ice-cold lemonade in the backyard would come to an end. All of those things Rita did so effortlessly to keep the house running smoothly and provide a loving atmosphere—things everyone had taken for granted for so many years—were coming undone. The house, and all of its order, was falling apart, and the ensuing chaos took the greatest toll on her husband, the ex-marine whose life had been so carefully regimented; Bob was also heavily burdened by the guilt of having cruelly blamed her for her weight gain, all the while having one foot out the door. Worse still, for him, was the realization that his children were about to lose the woman he describes as "their best friend," and during the holidays, no less. The building frustration, guilt, and sadness were understandably more than any man should have to bear, but his implicit reaction to this perfect storm of emotions would have devastating and lasting repercussions.

On Sunday, December 19, 1982, as his mother lay down the hall in the hospital bed delivered by hospice, Ed spent the wintry day inside, sitting in front of the television set, playing ATARI. Looking back, the only memory that could have clued him into the pending tragedy, had he paid greater attention, was an argument his father had with someone in the background of the day, but he was too wrapped up in his game to listen to what was being said. That evening, he put his video game on pause, went into the kitchen looking for something to eat, and managed to scrape out the last remains of dried-out peanut butter on to a piece of white Wonder bread. After slathering the whole thing with jelly, he returned to his game.

The realization that this might be Rita's last night on earth was just beginning to sink in for Bob when he walked into the kitchen and saw the jelly jar sitting open on the counter. Ed had no context for his father's rage. He didn't know his mother's life was about to expire nor that his father, who would later say, "She didn't deserve to die like that, it should have been me," was on the verge of emotional devastation. Nevertheless, that night, Rita's baby boy, Eddie, became the lightning rod for his father's anguish and despair.

"When he hit me, it just came out of the blue," Ed recalls. It's not that Ed was ever completely surprised by his father's temper, but most of the time it was just words. "A lot of times when my dad would scream," remembers Ed. "He'd throw things in the air and say terrible things, but that night, he came over and started kicking the ever-loving shit out of me. I had no idea what I did, or did not do, to deserve it." It would have been pointless to fight back or even run from his father, so Ed stood there and took the beating, trying not to cry and anger his father further. When it was all over, he did precisely what he was told to do; he went into the kitchen, put the lid back on the jelly jar, and went to bed, head severely throbbing from his father's violent outburst.

ED LAY AWAKE FOR A few hours, still petrified from what had just taken place that evening, but then he began to hear a painful groan coming from his mother's room, and he quietly, carefully, got out of bed, and headed down the hall. Ed stood frozen in the midnight shadows of the hallway across from his mother's room. His eleven-year-old mind knew instantly what his heart rejected. Listening to the gasp, the groan, and that final, unforgettable hiss of life as it escaped her lungs—he watched as his mother took her last breath. It would be years before he would tell anyone what he'd seen, and even longer before his father would accept the possibility that Ed's story could be true.

In the late hours of that December evening, just one week before Christmas, among the whispers of old ghosts living in the

Stoughton, Massachusetts, home—rumored to have once belonged to the cousin of Paul Revere—Ed shivered violently. In that moment, his entire life changed forever. In the recesses of his mind, he worried that his father might catch him out of bed, but as he wandered back to his bedroom, he was in shock over what he'd just witnessed.

It wasn't long before Ed heard the sudden rush of people coming and going outside his door. In a frenzy, his father told him to get up and get dressed, and then he was taken to the home of an aunt. No one *mentioned* his mother's death, and Ed feigned ignorance, still in shock from the physical and emotional trauma of the evening.

**TWO DAYS LATER, WHILE ED** was having a breakfast of Lender's bagels and cream cheese and hot tea, his father arrived to break the news of Rita's passing. Ed was taken by his father out of the kitchen into the den, where his dad said, "I've got something to tell you, son." But before he had a chance to speak, Ed looked up and said, "Dad, I know. Ma's not here anymore." Surprised, Bob assumed that Ed overheard a conversation, and he asked how he knew, but Ed refused to say anything else. In fact, it was the beginning of a silent treatment Bob would have to endure for a long time.

"Before his mom passed, he was always a quiet kid, always happy," recalls Bob. "But he was a really good kid—who wanted to spend time with me. We always watched movies together and things like that. But after her death, everything changed. I couldn't get him to do *anything*. He was shell shocked. He wouldn't talk to me, at all."

Even if Ed had the emotional capacity and the words to express what he had seen and what he was feeling, he didn't dare tell anyone; with the beating he had sustained for leaving the lid off a jelly jar, the consequences, he felt, of admitting that he had disobeyed his father by leaving his room and subsequently witnessing his mother's death were too great. He would carry this impossible secret, buried underneath the grief of extraordinary loss, for years to come, until he could no longer manage its profound effects.

**AT HIS MOTHER'S WAKE, ED** sat quietly in the back of the church, trying to figure it all out, as everyone else was busy dealing with his or her own individual grief. He had become an outsider, alone, left behind in the sorrow of his mother's wake, and his mind was filled with a mix of memories that he could not reconcile. At one point, as he stood in a line at the front of the room, greeting mourners with his family, he turned to look at his mother lying in the open casket and thought he saw a facial movement, a tic of some sort, indicating she was still alive. He watched her for a long time, hoping that her death was a mistake, and maybe that she was just sleeping, because she looked so peaceful and thin, as all of the fluid of her cancer-filled body was gone.

Ed, who had always been at the center of his mother's world, was now someone else's worry. He remembers family members scurrying around to find something of his to place in the casket, and they came up with a toy airplane. It should have been a *Star Wars* toy . . . that would have meant something. His mother would have understood the significance of that, but there was no one listening to him now.

Back at school, after Christmas break, Ed's friend Rudy didn't understand why Ed wasn't in class. Rudy had spent the holiday with family and didn't hear about Rita's death until the principal came in and made the announcement to the class. Rudy, whose own mother had died when he was in the first grade, had not only lost his neighborhood mother figure, but he greatly missed his best friend who would not return to school for a long time. When Ed did finally go back to school, his home life was so unsettled, he struggled to get through the rest of the year.

After Rita's death, everyone in the family seemed to scatter. While his older siblings were off living their lives as they had before his mother's death, his brother Tommy, with whom he shared a bedroom, went off and joined the service. Older sister Tami moved out of the house and into her own apartment down the road, while Deena, who is closest in age to Ed, withdrew into her own world and spent every night crying herself to sleep.

Ed spent a lot of time thinking about the fights and the harsh words that passed between his parents before his mother's death. He wondered if his dad—whom he describes as "disconnected" during the funeral, never crying once—even cared that his mother was gone. But then one night, as he passed outside the room where his father was packing up some of his mother's things, he was witness, once again, to a rare expression of his father's despair as the strong, proud marine broke down and wept.

Like most men of his generation, Bob did not take naturally to raising and nurturing children. It was something that women were supposed to do while men worked for a living. Now, without a wife, he was completely at a loss as to how to deal sensitively with his two youngest children. "I kept Christmas in the new room for them. I didn't know what else to do. I tried to talk to them, but I wasn't any good at it. They'd had a bomb unloaded on them. And then Eddie started to act strange, standing in the corner, talking to himself, all mumble-jumble," recalls Bob. "He would stand in the corner making strange noises, waving his arms, and grunting to himself. I didn't know what to do. I swear to God, I didn't." Before heading off to the service, Tommy remembers that Ed would lie in bed at night making the strange sounds in his sleep, and he knew something wasn't right.

As Ed's trauma over the loss of his mother continued to manifest itself in bizarre physical affectations, his inability to articulate his sorrow and pain created concern. "The problem is," says Ed, "nobody knew what I saw; only I knew. So they're thinking, 'poor kid, his mom just passed away, and he doesn't understand what's going on.' At that point, I not only understood what had happened, I had more going on inside of me—more emotions stirring—than anyone could possibly understand." The one person who would have understood was gone, and life was confusing. Ed was wrestling with many strange, new feelings and fears. "Suddenly, whenever I would get in the car with my sister to go do something fun," he recalls, "I felt like something bad was going to happen if we went a certain way or did a certain thing."

As the situation grew more desperate, and Bob's frustration increased, he made a decision that he thought was in the best interest of his children: he sent Eddie and his sister to live with his brother and sister-in-law. He hoped they would be better equipped to bring Eddie back to life than he would be on his own. But for Ed, being uprooted from his home, the place where the memories of his mother were alive, was devastating. It was also compounded by a certain fear. Even at his young age, he was trying to conceptualize death; the idea that his mother had gone to a place where Ed couldn't see or touch her was terrifying. He didn't want the same thing to happen to his dad. He wanted to stay by his side, be near to him, watch him to make sure nothing bad happened to him, even in spite of the jelly jar episode. Ed nevertheless yielded to his father's wishes, and the traumatized boy went to live with his aunt and uncle. "I didn't have the words to express myself, and what I was feeling," remembers Ed. "I could only do what I was told to do."

Ed may not have had the ability to express his thoughts and feelings aloud, but his deepest emotions rose up in silent expression as he related to the scenes of the movies and television shows he watched. He connected with story lines dealing with the issues of love, honor, and family, as they played out before him on the television set.

Ed recalls a specific moment during this time when he was visiting his auntie Queenie's house. Auntie Queenie was upstairs making his favorite chocolate and marshmallow candy, while downstairs he watched *Uncommon Valor* with his uncle "Crunch" Mac in their new entertainment room. "When you see moments like this on television, or in the movies—the love of a son, played by Patrick Swayze, for his father—those are *real* moments of emotion that live inside of us and stir us at the very core," Ed remembers. "I was raised on moments like that . . . television brought it out in me."

According to Ed's father, "not much changed" while Eddie lived with his aunt Betty and uncle Junior. And although Ed was drawn to Junior's strength and integrity and cites him as a role model for living a life of honor—being a man's man who meant what he said, who firmly believed in being truthful, and who never talked bad about anyone—it wasn't enough to erase the feelings of being so desperately unsettled. At the urging of Ed's older sister Tami, Bob took Ed to see a psychiatrist, hoping to find answers for his son's silence—but Ed refused to talk to the doctor.

In an attempt to bring his family back together and give Ed and his sister Deena a fresh start, Bob thought it would be a good idea to sell the house in Stoughton and make a permanent move to their summer home on Cape Cod. It was not a discussion he had with his children; he just did it. Suddenly, inexplicably, Ed was taken to live in a world far away from the smell of spring lilacs outside his window, the tire swing hanging from the tall tree in the backyard, and his best friend, Rudy. It was the only home he'd ever known—the refuge he associated with his mother's love and protection. As he watched his dad load boxes into a U-Haul to take to their summer home, Ed had no idea he was leaving his childhood home forever, and he was never given a chance to say good-bye to it.

Time just kept moving forward, and the changes it inflicted upon him were too many, and too fast. He wanted it all to stop. He wanted to turn back time and make everything the way it was. He wanted to stay in the one place where his mother lived in his heart and mind, but it had all vanished in the rearview window of his father's car as they left Stoughton for the last time.

**THE HOUSE ON THE CAPE** was a brand-new raised ranch with all the modern conveniences. It didn't have a long history, or rumors of ghosts. It didn't smell like an antique store. There wasn't even a hint of his mother's shampoo freshness or the lingering scent of cigarettes she smoked at the kitchen table while playing her games.

Other than Ed's sister Deena and his grandmother Sitto—who temporarily acted as their caretaker—and of course the television, the house was a vast, unfamiliar, five-bedroom emptiness. The joy that Ed once got from playing outside was gone. The scenery was foreign, and he had no friends in the neighborhood to play with. He missed Rudy, he missed the tree swing, he missed the swimming pool. So he retreated inside to live among the things he could touch, that had once been touched by his mother. He began to seek comfort in the physical objects, the toy Transformers, GI Joes, the Star Wars figures, and the Darth Vader costume his mother bought him, all of which had a calming effect on his mind. He would curl up on the sofa, watch his usual cartoons and television programs, and relish in the familiarity of it all, reliving the warm and cozy feelings from the childhood that felt a million miles away. The toys and television had become Ed's mental catharsis.

When Tommy came home from the service, he would come by to help Bob get the kids off to school. He recalls it was hard to get Ed moving in the morning. "The harder I pushed, the longer it took for Ed to get his things together and make his way to the car," says Tommy. Ed, he reports, was always going back to check and recheck things he needed to bring to school, and touch certain things before he could move out the door. "Looking back," recalls Tom, "it was Ed's OCD starting to reveal itself. It wasn't because Ed was lazy, but we didn't know that at the time."

A self-described "geek," Ed was the skinny new kid, in a new environment, and he became the target of the neighborhood bullies. He wasn't comfortable at school, he wasn't completely comfortable at home, and by the time he hit thirteen, he wasn't comfortable in his own body. "I was trying to become an adult and deal with the fact that my mom wasn't there, and there was no one in the family for me to talk to about adolescence." Emotionally, Ed says he continued to identify closely with the young kid inside himself and still enjoyed his cartoons and toys in spite of the growing pressures of being a teenager. And while Ed wasn't as close to his father as he had been as a child, there was a constant undercurrent of worry in his life that he, too, might die. His dad wasn't home much, but Ed always made it a point to know where his father was, checking in on him to make sure he was okay. Life was confusing, and he admits, "I lived a lonely, motherf'ing life, always asking myself, 'What the hell about me?'"

Ed says that he quickly realized that his survival, and gathering friends and family around him, depended on his personality. "Being a sweet, geeky, book-smart kid helped me make friends," says Ed. Ed's attachment to his friends was intense and loyal. The more preoccupied he became with his friendships, the more he was distracted from the constant thought of dealing with the loss of his mother. "I didn't get closure to the problem and never developed the coping skills I needed, but I felt I was honoring her by *trying* to be happy," says Ed.

**BY THE TIME HIGH SCHOOL** rolled around, Ed had grown into a tall, good-looking teenager. Tommy, who had always been a terrific athlete, encouraged Ed to get involved in sports. Ed never considered himself a jock at 140 pounds, but he managed to make the football team in his junior and senior years. By this time, Ed had naturally developed a quick wit that made him popular with his friends, and he had become part of a small group of guys. Kevin Frye, tri-captain of the Falmouth High School football team, and one of Ed's closest friends, remembers, "Eddie would always go above and beyond to help his friends out, and he wanted everybody around him to be happy. We all knew he didn't have much of a home life, he and his dad were not the closest, so his friends pretty much became his family."

No one ever really talked about the fact that Ed's mother died, but his friends all knew, and there were times when Ed would become suddenly pensive. When someone would ask, "What's up, Eddie?" he would simply tell them he had a lot of things on his mind. It was clear these sporadic interruptions in his otherwise upbeat mood reflected much deeper issues. Kevin remembers times when it would be hard for Ed to go home after they'd been hanging out together because he really had nothing to go home to but an empty house.

Ed's high school football career was unremarkable. He was tall, but skinny and not by *any* stretch the most physically gifted athlete on the field, and his playing time was usually limited to the few minutes at the end of the fourth quarter. Ed may not have seen a lot of game time, but he remembers overhearing one of his coaches say, "the kid's got a lot of heart," and that made him feel good. But even when he *did* play, there was rarely anyone around to watch who could later pat him on the back and offer words of encouragement. The only reason he played football, he now admits, is that he wanted to make his brother, Tom, proud.

Tom would show up at practice whenever he was in town, but Ed's dad was always too busy working to come to his games. Ed says he never pressured him about it because he figured work was something his father did to bury the feelings he had for Ed's mother. In the back of his mind, though, he always knew that if his mother were alive, she would have been sitting in the grandstands at every game, supporting him even on days when he did nothing more than warm the bench. It was the "what might have been" that was a constant source of heartache and sadness in Ed's life. On Thanksgiving Day 1989, which marked the last game of Ed's senior year, when Bob did finally show up with Tom to watch him play, there was another heartbreaking turn of events. Ed was sidelined for the entire game. His dad never got to see him play.

When he wasn't out with his buddies, Ed found solace in the soft glow of his television set in the basement, but it was the VCR that changed his experience in a whole new way as he watched his favorite television shows and movies over and over again, hitting the rewind button as often as he chose, dissecting and analyzing the actions and reactions of his favorite scenes and characters. If he watched a tape and caught someone saying the word *death,* or what Ed calls the "d-word,"—he would rewind it so they would repeat it an even number of times, because if something was said an even number of times, it was like an "eraser to a chalkboard"—it simply disappeared. If he saw something he didn't like, he would fast-forward past the scene to "wash it out." He says he would always time it perfectly, because he could "feel" it, before hitting play again.

Rewinding gave Ed complete control of time within his movie and television world, and gradually between 1992 and 1995, he would transition his power from a videotape process to a mental and physical process that would completely consume him.

**FOR THE NEXT SEVERAL YEARS,** Ed continued to suppress the painful secret of his mother's last moments, but as he watched his heroes on television, he made a conscious decision that he would live his life like a movie. *He* would become a hero, too. The idea that someone would be willing to lay down his life for another human being resonated deeply within him. As a child, he wasn't able to save his mother, but as a man, he would find a way to save the rest of the people he loved.

*I dreamt my dreams forwards and backwards.*

—ED ZINE

# CHAPTER 3

# Time Equals Progression, Progression Equals Death

◀◀

TIMES WERE TOUGH IN NEW England. In 1990, banks up
and down the eastern seaboard were closing as the real estate
market collapsed, sending the economy into a free fall. For guys
like Ed's dad working in the construction business, the pressure
of the recession was unrelenting. Tensions ran high all around,
and dreams of big fortunes degenerated into modest quests for
survival.

But Ed was a dreamer. A year out of high school, he still believed his mother's prediction that he was destined for something
special, and he wasn't prepared to accept the status quo. He was
a talented, self-taught artist who'd done his first oil painting at
the age of four, and drawing became his passion. Without sup-

port and direction, however, Ed didn't have any idea what to do with his talent. His dad didn't think of art as a "real" job, so Ed floundered—doing odds-and-ends jobs for his dad in the plumbing business, yet fighting the pressure to make the family business a full-time career. The rest of the time, he locked himself up in the basement and watched television, in part to contemplate his future, but mostly because of the deep feeling of loss that consumed him when his friends left for college.

**"DO SOMETHING, OR GET THE** hell out of my house." It wasn't easy trying to figure out one's life goal under the constant pressure of a threat, but it was the only way that Ed's father knew how to motivate. Pushing and prodding is what worked for Bob when he was in the U.S. Marines, and threats worked in the rough-and-tumble world of construction, but Ed was programmed differently. As a child, he was taught by his mother to respond to gentle, loving, nurturing support and direction. He didn't respond well to Bob's tough-love approach and was quickly becoming immobilized by anxiety.

Ed's childhood friend, Rudy Harris, was off at college living his own dream as a starting fullback for the Clemson University Tigers. After Ed and his family moved to Cape Cod, Rudy became somewhat of a local celebrity as the star player for the Brockton High School football team, the number one high school team in the country in 1989. Years later, Rudy would wonder how Ed's life might have been different had he been able to stay in Stoughton and Rudy and Ed had been allowed to grow up together. Each of them understood what it was like to lose a mother so young, and with his family frequently absent, Ed perhaps could've benefited from Rudy's "older brother" compassion and positive attitude if he had been a constant presence. Maybe Ed, too, would have developed as a star athlete.

As it was, the two continued their long-distance friendship through their high school years. Ed spent a lot of time riding the bench for his high school team while Rudy went on to become the top running back in the state. There wasn't a high school football player in Massachusetts who didn't know the name Rudy Harris, and Ed was proud of his childhood friend.

IN THE FALL OF 1990, tired of his loneliness, Ed spontaneously decided to visit Rudy down at Clemson. After the fourteen-hour ride, Ed pulled his car up to just a few blocks from the school and made his way across campus to Rudy's residence hall. The sun was shining, the weather was crisp, and there was an air of excitement. As Ed looked around at the happy faces of students, he could feel the anxiety of his life melt away.

Ed had no specific time plan for his visit, but he quickly became known as "Rudy's boy from back east." With this acceptance by members of the football crew, which at Clemson, a perennial Division One contender, *meant* something, he enjoyed the vicarious thrill of watching his childhood friend practice each day from the sideline.

One afternoon, while casually tossing the ball back and forth with Rudy along the perimeter of the Clemson practice field after one of the team's workouts, as Ed imagined how proud his mother would have been to see him play college football alongside Rudy, he remembers being stopped by the head strength coach for the Tigers, Gary Wade. Wade, who seemed to take notice of some zip in those relaxed tosses, asked Ed where he played his high school football.

Ed was a scrawny guy in high school who had a lot of heart, but who never really spent much time on the radar of his coaches. Now, according to Rudy, a Clemson coach was taking notice of Ed.

Ed says he followed Coach Wade to the Jervey Athletic Center and that on the way there they spoke about what it would take for him to be considered for the Tigers football squad. "I felt Coach Wade recognized in me something that he saw in the athletes who were full-scale recruits and Division One starters," says Ed. "He invested the time in me to make me feel positive and made me feel that I had the ability to find greatness within myself."

This trip to escape the confines of his father's basement had suddenly turned into a new lease on life for Ed. The prospect of attending Clemson as a student athlete sounds like a long shot for a guy already one year out of high school who'd never even started in a *high school* game. But even though he was a lithe 140 pounds, Ed knew his six-feet, two-inch frame could handle the added bulk he needed to put on in order to play. The biggest obstacle, as Ed saw it, was not so much the athletic component, but the additional requirements for Clemson's stringent admission process.

Regardless, he placed his faith in his mother's prescience, and his resolve was strong. And with a copy of Coach Wade's workout routine in hand, Ed returned home to Cape Cod, dream in tow, ready to fulfill the commitment he made to himself to one day play for the Clemson Tigers. But within days of coming home after that promising trip to South Carolina, and making that pronouncement to family and friends, his anxiety returned—it was the kind of anxiety he experienced when he was young—that nagging feeling that something bad would happen if he made the wrong directional choice while driving or walking.

Dividers in roads caused overwhelming stress, and Ed would plan his daily travels to avoid them. He was panic-stricken by the thought of going around a one-way rotary, which is very common in his home state of Massachusetts, without being able to reverse the turn. None of it made sense to him, and he didn't understand why doing any of these things seemed so ominous, but they did.

Ed would soon take multimile detours to avoid rotaries. Not only did these episodes inconvenience and frustrate him, they of course proved trying to his passengers. Friends would often take the wheel and suggest that Ed, sitting in the front passenger seat, close his eyes while they executed turns. But it didn't matter whether his eyes were open or closed, his body had its own sensors that would sound off in his brain, like a thousand sharp fingernails shrieking down a chalkboard. This was accompanied by the foreboding feeling that if he didn't follow his mind's directive, something terrible would happen; specifically, something bad might happen to someone he loved. It was the same foreboding feeling he first had when his older sister and aunts would try and push him and Deena to go out to do "fun stuff" as their mother lay dying at home. His mind tried to adjust to the intuitive notion that he had to correct the situation with an opposite reaction, and the fear created by these peculiar, intrusive thoughts was relieved only when he followed an action that his body and mind "felt" was correct.

The only way to placate his torturous anxiety was to insist on being let out before they reached the rotary so he could walk a straight line through it and then meet the car on the other side. His friends thought he was acting crazy, and they ridiculed his behavior. Ed was confused and embarrassed by his illogical behavior, which, in turn, compounded the anxiety and escalated his cycle of obsessive thinking and compulsive reaction. As is often the case with OCD, the disorder was actually feeding on itself to grow stronger.

Although one might logically assume that the obsessive-compulsive disorder slowly and steadily gaining a foothold in Ed's mind was triggered by the stress of his new athletic and intellectual pursuits, he doesn't remember feeling particularly nervous about making a bid for Clemson. What he felt was the uncontrollable worry of something happening to, say, his father if Ed walked the wrong way or touched something incorrectly—for example, if he touched his index finger to his middle finger and then failed to retouch it the same way an even number of times. It was the *guilt* that he felt . . . the pressure of "what if." What if something happened to his father in a rare moment when Ed was carefree, and not constantly worrying? If he wasn't maintaining the rituals within rituals of touching and going the right way, he would be responsible for whatever unfortunate event that might take place.

But Ed dug deep within himself and pressed on to reach that goal of the great thing he was meant to do with his life. If he could just join his friend Rudy at Clemson, he knew everything would be okay.

THE GUYS AT ED'S GYM comprised a group of mostly blue-collar workers living in the rugged world of construction. When Ed showed up at the gym immediately following his trip, telling everybody that he wholly aspired to play for Clemson—at quarterback, no less—the guys rolled their eyes, thinking him crazy for reasons completely unrelated to the OCD, which, at that point in time, hadn't yet manifested itself during Ed's workouts. The consensus among them was that Ed's pursuit was a pipe dream. They started to call Ed, "Martin Luther King, the man with the dream." But Phil Miller—a Georgetown graduate and former college athlete who owned a construction company—had compassion for the starry-eyed kid:

"Back then, Eddie wasn't a standout athlete, but he was a standout person. While all the guys teased him, Ed stayed focused, relentless in his workout. Everyone watched as he loaded up ridiculous amounts of weights on the machine, doing endless repetitions, and doing so many squats every night that his muscles started splitting his pants wide open. He would be the last one working out in the gym every night, telling everyone else, 'just one more set.' He was determined to prove everybody wrong."

Ed put himself in the zone. He drank weight-gaining shakes, took Metrx and EAS supplements, religiously ate a pound of pasta every night, and strictly followed Coach Wade's workout regimen: chest and legs on Mondays and Thursdays; shoulders, back, and arms on Tuesdays and Fridays. He also developed his own system of sprints, which he ran in the evenings at a secluded spot on the heights overlooking the water. He would throw a football roughly twenty yards out in front of him, sprint to it, pick it up, and throw it twenty more; he repeated this routine over and over for hours on end, always in solitude.

One day, his gym buddy Phil volunteered to practice out in the parking lot of the gym after they finished their workouts. It was meant as a friendly gesture, but he was genuinely impressed by Ed's arm. "He starts zinging the ball across the parking lot," recalls

Phil, "and I was like, 'Wow, this kid has some real talent. *Especially* for somebody who wasn't a starter in high school.'" Phil couldn't really say whether his young friend would be successful in getting past the Clemson admissions process, let alone play for the Tigers, but given Ed's enthusiasm, Phil wouldn't count him out.

Within five months, all of Ed's training and discipline paid off as he packed on 45 pounds of sheer muscle, bringing his weight to a viable 185 pounds. But rather than invoking the admiration of the doubters at the gym, Ed's altered physique and increased strength changed the snide comments to earnest scrutiny. Ed became understandably defensive and even expressed his willingness to submit himself to blood and urine tests to prove his progress was legitimate.

Drug related it wasn't, but there are many who now believe that it may have been Ed's underlying OCD, and the nature of his relentless obsessions, driving him toward perfection.

Regardless of the role Ed's then undiagnosed condition might have played in his seemingly instant success, his drive to do the extraordinary took on an added dimension. Honoring his mother was of course a primary motivator, but being surrounded by skeptics placed a new value on the unconditional faith he believed Coach Wade had placed in him, and he resolved to do him proud.

In January 1991, although he was still ineligible academically, Ed was ready to head back to Clemson. He needed to be in a positive atmosphere, where Rudy and all the guys could take in his progress. He wanted his adopted mentor, Coach Wade, to see for himself what Ed was capable of accomplishing in such a short period of time. At a time when Ed needed it most, he received the positive reinforcement he sought. "Coach Wade has a way of making you believe in something great," remembers Ed, "and that you can conquer the world. He is all about mind, spirit, and soul, and what defines you as a human being. He said he was preparing me for the biggest game: life."

Ed was now ready to take the next step toward his goal of becoming part of the Clemson family and, upon his return home to Cape Cod, he immediately enrolled in classes at the local community college to meet that academic requirement.

**IT WAS JUST SO LOFTY** a goal, and as many friends and family members stood back and watched skeptically, there were a few, like Phil and Ed's sister Tami, who hoped that this was the beginning of something big for Ed. But the guys at the gym were still pretty relentless in their caustic remarks. Intellectually, Ed understood it was an implausible dream that was hard for people to understand, and he turned the negativity into motivation to keep him pushing harder.

The truth is that Ed had never really wanted to play football. Art was his true passion; however, his dad didn't see this as a real career choice—and whenever Ed brought it up, his dad would remind him of the stigma of "starving artists." But Ed couldn't ignore the feeling of being important and respected by simply working out alongside the team when he was at Clemson. "I was still trying to find that great thing," remembers Ed. "I was doing the mental Google search for my future career and thought maybe this was it." Beneath the surface, though, lay that chronic anxiety that felt like an annoying undercurrent of electricity in his brain humming day and night that he couldn't turn off, like a severe case of tinnitus. More and more, he would find himself hesitating before he could move forward, needing to retrace his steps or read words forward and backward to try and correct the discomfort; but the mental and physical hiccups, the hesitation that kept him from moving steadily forward, was something he could not shut down.

All stress in Ed's life, even that caused by something as ordinary as his friends leaving for school, or his indecision about his future, led him straight into the painful memory of his mother's death. Ed's emotional foundation was broken. He'd never reconciled his mother's death in any way, and without that closure, the added demand of having to prove himself academically before he could even *consider* applying to Clemson was creating further instability. It wasn't only the work itself; just getting to class at the community college became an enormous challenge. He found himself avoiding certain routes to school, making detours to retrace the journey back and forth dozens of times until he felt comfortable enough to continue.

But when he finally got to class, his preoccupations began to affect his ability to absorb information, and even his literacy. He found himself stuck on pages, reading the sentences over and over again, trying to process information. It could take him several hours to complete an assignment of just a few pages. He began to feel the need to read every sentence forward *and* backward, repeatedly, until his mind was fully satisfied.

It was the same for road signs when he traveled to class. He *had* to read them forward and backward, or he didn't feel comfortable enough to keep driving. School was less than twenty miles away, and yet the journey could take him several hours. He would become physically exhausted and ill just *thinking* about the trip to school and, as a result, he often wouldn't go. And all the while Ed had no idea what was happening to him.

Not surprisingly, his growing obsessions were becoming more and more difficult to conceal. If he happened to ride to the local McDonald's, and his friends were driving, he would ask to be let out of the car before they went through the drive-through. He would then walk ahead and wait for them to circle around with the car to go back out the exit. He would explain it to his friends by saying he just wanted to "take a walk," but when this started happening on a regular basis, the guys started teasing him about his quirky behavior.

As his compulsions grew, in order to address the demands of what he would later find out was OCD, Ed began offering to drive whenever he went out with friends. He could no longer simply take a left turn into the parking lot of a local restaurant. He would have to drive all the way around the block and come in from the other side so he could take a right turn. Left turns were considered odd and right turns were considered even. His mind rejected anything odd, and if he took a left turn, it didn't "feel" right. "It would drive us nuts!" remembers high school buddy Kevin Frye. "We'd go, 'what in the hell are you doing, Eddie?' but he would either ignore us, or say, 'I just *want* to go this way, that's all.'"

On any given day, Ed would obsessively tiptoe across tile floors, maneuvering his size-twelve feet into the center of each square, trying to avoid the cracks of grout between each one. This child's game, for Ed, was a deadly serious endeavor to avoid touching the lines for fear that something truly catastrophic would happen to someone he loved.

IN 1992, ED HAD NO idea he had OCD, but he knew there was something different about his thinking process and his need to do things a certain way. Seeking medical help wasn't even a consideration, however, because, to Ed, *thinking differently* didn't constitute an illness. He was putting himself under a lot of pressure to try and make a bid for Clemson, and he didn't have many cheerleaders to support him, so he decided to get away—head back to South Carolina where everything seemed brighter, and he, ostensibly, had a plan. On his own, he decided he would take the classes he needed to fulfill Clemson's academic requirements for admission locally, then enroll as a full-time Clemson student, make the team, and play the following year.

But to start, Ed figured that if he showed up at the athletic center every day with his buddies to attend team workouts, he would continue to be noticed and evaluated in a positive light, and he would prove his value as a potential member of the team.

He certainly wasn't disappointed on his arrival. He says Rudy, Coach Wade, and the guys on the team seemed happy to see him, and they acknowledged his dramatic physical change. His plan was to crash in the dorm with his buddy while he tried to get classes worked out at the local community college, and hang out with the team as much as possible. And since Rudy carried a lot of weight as one of the Tigers' star players, Ed was given more latitude to hang out on the sidelines during practice and occasionally throw the ball around with the other players.

"Not everybody liked him being on the field," says Rudy, who would later go on to play briefly in the NFL for the Tampa Bay Buccaneers and the Washington Redskins, referring to the coaching staff. "But we'd put on our pads, and he would be out there throwing the ball with us. He had a great arm, and the coaches were watching him."

Rudy knew Ed was still struggling emotionally with the loss of his mother, and he regretted the fact that he hadn't been around to help him through it when they were "like brothers" growing up in Stoughton, so he was determined to use the small amount of influence he held within the Clemson football program to help Ed get a shot as a walk-on the following year. But he knew it was a long shot. "I was trying my best to help Ed, but it's really hard to play as part of the team if you're not there on scholarship."

If nothing else, Ed is persistent, so, regardless of his unofficial student status, Ed was practicing with the team and hanging out with the players after practice was over, and he would use every opportunity he could to spend time talking to Coach Wade. But no matter how much access he was granted, or how many heartwarming conversations he had with Wade, there would be no happy ending to Ed's story—not at Clemson, at least. As the OCD quickly metastasized, unbeknownst to Ed, he found himself unable to attend the local community college, where he was trying to earn grades Clemson would find admissible.

**WITH INCREASING FREQUENCY, ED WOULD** see flashes of himself as a young boy, standing in the hallway, watching his mother pass, and be so consumed that he found it hard to concentrate. And these visions led to his incrementally intensifying obsession with protecting his father, who was healthy and happy living back in Cape Cod, from harm.

The ominous turning point came one day as he walked across campus from the dorm to the athletic field. He came to a fork in the path and was suddenly gripped by an overwhelming fear when he looked to the left—which was odd, and bad in his mind—and visualized the image of a skull and crossbones, and panicked. He froze in place, shook his head, and looked to the right of the path, at which point he had mental flashes—images of his father getting killed in a terrible car accident. Back and forth, he looked at the two places where he could step forward, but the images were the same; left—skull and crossbones, right—fatal accident. He couldn't move, stricken with terror that if he stepped forward, even an inch, someone would die.

These vague, unsettling *feelings* of OCD, and the harrowing moments when nothing feels right, defy logical explanation. They come in varying degrees to people who have the disorder, and in Ed's case they were extraordinary and severe. But the torment in not knowing *why* the thoughts are occurring, and the fact that there is nothing tangible on which to hang the agony born from intrusive thoughts, is sheer anguish.

Ed remembers standing helplessly frozen in place, for more than two hours, in the path of a rush of students forced to detour around him as they headed to class. The embarrassment of not being able to move away from the crowd was dwarfed by the terror that any move he made had the potential to impact the life of his father.

"OCD is like having your head in a vice . . . it keeps cranking and turning, getting tighter, and tighter, and the only way to relieve it is to do its bidding," says Ed. "At the same time, you're rejecting the thought process because you *want* to function properly."

Closing his eyes, and rocking back and forth, trying to soothe the wild beasts in his mind, Ed began trying to think of happier moments to distract himself from the painful vision that consumed him, and the humiliation of standing statuelike in the middle of campus. He finally became "unlocked," he says, by thinking of *Star Wars* and recalling the first time he saw *The Empire Strikes*

*Back* with his father. Ed seized that fleeting moment, turned around, ran back the way he came to find a pay phone and call his father to confirm that he'd made the right decision.

Bob knew Ed's concern over his health and well-being through the years was extraordinary, but he remained sympathetic in this because he knew it stemmed from the loss of his mother. Still, this call was a signal to him that things were not going as smoothly as he hoped they would, and he worried about what Ed's next step would be if Clemson didn't work out.

Of course he found his father was alive and well, so Ed returned to the dorm where he was staying with friends and collapsed on his bed. The strain of carrying what he thought was his father's welfare on his shoulders for those two hours left Ed in such physical and emotional distress that he spent the next three days in bed with a migraine headache.

"Logically, I *knew* that the odds of anything bad happening to my father are slim," says Ed with regard to his OCD mind. "But if I walk to the left, instead of walking to the right, and something *does* happen to my father, I am responsible for his death. I will, in essence, have killed him."

When Ed complied with OCD's demand to move right, left, or not at all, he was momentarily relieved from the anxiety caused by his obsession with his father's safety, or whomever else is on his mind—his brother or his sisters. Ed equates this adrenaline rush of relief to the hero of a movie who has just saved someone from impending death. It is a surge that by the pure nature of OCD simply reinforced the cycle, and giving in to his anxiety meant Ed was reinforcing the cycle. The more he indulged these sorts of compulsions to get relief from the obsessions of OCD, the greater the intensity of OCD's demands.

CHAPTER 4

# Time to Go Home

◀◀

ED KNEW IT WAS TIME to go home. He could no longer handle the stress of getting everything together academically to
make the bid to Clemson, and he continued to be consumed with
worry that something bad would happen to his father. When Ed
returned home to Cape Cod, he remembers how angry his father
was that he had not been successful. It was devastating for Ed
to have to admit to his dad, a man who'd spent half his teenage
years as a marine in wartime, that he didn't understand what was
happening to him, making him unable to continue.

But Bob doesn't recall himself expressing or even feeling any
such anger. In fact, he suggests that Ed was just on overdrive,
setting himself up for disappointment by expecting too much. "I

think he just overburdened himself by trying to do too much," remembers Bob. "Eddie went off the deep end."

Bob tried putting his son to work in the plumbing business with him, but the two fought vociferously during the rides to work together. "I would drive and when we'd get to the rotaries, Eddie would say, 'Dad, let me out here.'" When Bob refused, Ed would start yelling, "Let me out. Let me out!" Recalling that frustrating time, Bob says, "I wondered what the hell was wrong with him." Over time, as Ed's condition got progressively worse, Bob says, "A short ride anywhere with Eddie could turn into a six-hour trip."

It's not that Ed's "quirks" hadn't been noticed on occasion by the rest of the family, but for lack of understanding, or severity, they'd been dismissed. But by 1992, his symptoms, although still lacking an official diagnosis of OCD, were hard to ignore.

Periodically, whenever the entire Zine family would gather upstairs for holidays or birthdays, they couldn't help but notice Ed was becoming more and more withdrawn. To Ed, avoiding people, even the family he loved so very much, was the least painful way for him to deal with whatever strange affliction now tormented him. He struggled to hide his embarrassing ritual of having to walk backward down the steps, and doing it multiple times until it *felt* right; often he would simply remain downstairs until everyone left. Ed's older sister Tami remembers watching in disbelief the first time she witnessed Ed walking up the stairs backward when he didn't think anyone was watching. She didn't understand what she was seeing, but knew this signaled a much bigger problem than anyone had previously imagined. At this point, though, she kept it to herself and simply hoped it would go away.

**THE EMOTIONAL PAIN OF OCD** isn't limited to personal, internal obsessions unique to the sufferer. OCD sufferers often become inordinately concerned with *external* events. In Ed's case, it was the Persian Gulf War. He listened to reports on television and became consumed with the fear that his brother, Tom, who was serving in the army, would be called overseas—and killed. Although this is a normal concern for any military family member, the anxiety that it triggered in Ed resulted in an exaggerated cycle of obsessive worrying, and a growing compulsion to keep "things" in place—a combination of "just right" obsessions and hoarding—that began to erupt on a greater scale. If, for example, a hat was sitting atop the television when Ed heard something on TV that inspired him to feel good—someone won something, a life was saved, or he saw an inspirational ending to a movie—the hat couldn't be moved—it had to stay in that place, never to be moved, and as long as it did, nothing bad would happen to Tom.

Contamination fears are probably the most well-known symptom of OCD and can be triggered when an OCD sufferer encounters illness. For Ed, the obsession with germs fully manifested itself in September of 1993, when HBO premiered the groundbreaking movie *And the Band Played On,* a dramatic story about the evolution of the AIDS crisis.

Ed acutely remembers this film, as well as an urban legend originating around the same time about a guy in New York City who wakes up after a one-night stand, and on his mirror, written in lipstick, are the words, "Welcome to the AIDS club." This absurd, perverted horror story caused Ed to obsessively worry about contracting HIV. Ed's OCD mind had equated sex with AIDS and he began to fear sexual contact. Although Ed had never been promiscuous, OCD turned his decision to practice abstinence until he found the girl he was going to marry into avoidance of all human contact within a year.

INCREASINGLY, OCD ALTERED ED'S PHYSICAL reality. Once, when a stranger accidentally bumped into him, he followed him a short distance and carefully maneuvered a way to gently bump his arm back, without being noticed, so the event was erased in his mind.

As the manifestation of OCD symptoms increased, Ed became profoundly aware of the physical space around him. If anyone walked behind him, or parked a car behind his car, he would feel trapped—as if bound by an invisible rope that he couldn't break—preventing him from rewinding his steps and actions so that he could properly erase them in time. His older sister Tami recalls that when he rode in her car, she would have to park in a place where no one could park behind her, so he would not get "trapped."

And so much as *hearing* the word *death,* or any variation of it, would instantly stunt his thought process and even his ability to move, sending him into a state of sheer panic. His heart races, he gets hot flashes, he begins to sweat, and he even struggles to breathe. He suffers extreme flashbacks and he is instantly transported back to the night of his mother's death, which becomes as vivid to him as it was when he was eleven years old. The only way he can logistically and calmly process any variation of the words *death, dead, or die* is to spell them out, or ask *others* to spell them out, instead of verbalizing them in conversation. If someone who is unaware of his need to have the word spelled out says it unwittingly, he has to have them repeat it, so it is "erased." Eventually, he came up with a word that he could tolerate for death: "freath."

**IN JANUARY 1993, IN SPITE** of the mysterious and ever-increasing symptoms that plagued him, Ed loaded up his car and his dog, Zeus, and, with his father in the driver's seat, made the fourteen-hour trip to South Carolina one last time. Ed was desperately unhappy trying to work in construction with his father and dealing with the mix of intrusive thoughts, the counting and checking rituals, and the constant worry that plagued him. He hoped the incident at the path fork on campus was a fluke and that a change in scenery would now do him good. He hoped that being around Rudy and the guys, who had made him feel so welcome, and simply throwing the football around, could perhaps empower him again. Bob was at a total loss as to how to help his son find his way in life, and he hoped that going back to Clemson would help.

But the moment his father left and headed to the train station to go back home, after helping Ed get set up at a local hotel, Ed curled up on his bed. Like so many people with OCD, he was lost. He didn't understand how everyone else could be so carefree when his entire world was fraught with worry of every kind. Though Bob was out of sight, he was hardly out of mind, as Ed now believed that he held the key to his father's life in his every move.

Of course recapturing the good feeling he once had at Clemson was out of the question. He called Rudy, but he couldn't commit to plans that involved leaving the room. He remembers one of the guys from the team, Brad Thompson, stopping by to see him, but Ed never managed to make his way back to campus. And after spending two weeks mostly watching television, ordering food, taking Zeus outside for brief walks—he packed up his car and went home.

Back home at his father's house, Ed could only motivate himself to work sporadically, and only insofar as he wanted to ensure his father's safety. He would carry all of the heavy tools and equipment up and down the stairs because he didn't want to risk Bob getting hurt. His activities became increasingly more limited, to the point where he was staying in the basement watching movies and cartoons and playing video games nearly full-time. When he *did* venture out to someplace like the local mall, one trip would turn into a series of subsequent trips throughout the week, as many as sixteen times back and forth, to erase the initial excursion as if it never happened.

Rewinding and erasing an event in Ed's mind meant that one action—whatever it was—moved him forward in time, and doing it again precisely in an even number that felt right to him, erased the first action and thus kept time in its place—at least in *his* mind. There is absolutely nothing logical about this way of thinking. And there is no clinical explanation for Ed's specific rewinding manifestation—that is, his *obsession* over the number of times something happened being connected to time in his mind and his *compulsion* to erase the event by repeating the ritual to, in his mind, keep time from moving forward. Obsessions and compulsions manifest differently in every patient.

Between his last visit to Clemson in 1993 and the summer of 1995, there were periods of time when the severity of Ed's OCD seemed to wane before rebounding into greater obsessive and compulsive rituals. Tom came home from the service, bringing with him a sense of calm and relief and giving Ed a greater sense of family. Life was far from perfect for Ed, but now it was at least manageable and ordinary. But OCD was the dark shadow lurking in the corner—it never completely went away—and every time it showed its face, it became harder to dismiss.

High school friend Jason Peters recalls a trip with Ed to Emerald Square City Mall in North Attleboro, about an hour and a half from home. Ed seemed fine the whole day, until he accidentally dropped his keys in the mall's parking lot as the two were about to head home. The slippage was simple enough, but when Ed reached down to pick them up, his hand brushed the ground. This started a chain reaction of touching obsessions, and the need to touch and retouch the parking lot an even number of times to erase the event.

Ed didn't want to inconvenience Jason, or embarrass himself, and he fought the desperate urge to continue touching the ground, though he hadn't reached that elusive magic number of touches that *felt right,* and forced himself to get back into the car. He remained quiet on the way home as he counted backward and forward, visualizing his hand touching the ground, hoping this would satiate his seemingly uncontrollable mental demands. But halfway home, Ed succumbed to the anguish that plagued him, and told Jason to turn back—he didn't tell him the real reason because that would've been humiliating; instead he said he'd dropped his driver's license back at the parking lot at the same time he'd dropped his keys, and he had to go back to get it.

Jason turned the car around, and when they returned to the spot, Ed got out of the car and began acting as if he were frantically searching for his license, while he touched the spot in the parking lot over and over until he reached the number of touches, even of course, that would placate the anxiety The number was always different, so he could be in one spot for four minutes, or four hours. Fortunately, he was able to accomplish the touches he needed to make in just a couple of minutes as he "frantically searched" for his driver's license. It wasn't until years later that Ed admitted the ruse to Jason.

**THE NEED TO WALK BACKWARD** and retrace his steps was becoming much harder to suppress, and consequently more difficult to hide. "We'd go into public places and Eddie would have to walk down the stairs backwards," recalls Jason. "It got pretty bad. I had an idea what was going on because I had seen a television special about OCD, but the other guys just thought he was acting crazy and would make fun of him." Jason recalls some of their friends doing impersonations of Ed's behavior when he wasn't around, mimicking the backward walking and tiptoeing across tiles. They weren't being malicious, he says, they were just young guys having fun; but when Ed's rituals started to include wearing the same clothes over and over, which of course he couldn't even *attempt* to hide, they teased him about it to his face.

**IN 1995, ED INVITED KEVIN** Frye's cousin Donald to live with him when he needed a place to stay. Ed thought it might be good for him to have the company, and he hoped it would be a distraction from his repetitive behaviors. But the OCD had already created in him the need to manage the perfect placement of everything in his world. It didn't matter if it was a bar of soap, a magazine on the table, or a box on the floor. His world was already becoming an "OCD Holy Ground," and the meticulousness with which he monitored his belongings—protective over them as if they were his children, not wanting them moved, or so much as *touched*—was extraordinary. "I can look at the markings and placement of things, and I can see within millimeters if something has been moved," says Ed.

In the bathroom, Ed would look at the seams of the tile, gauge the gap between the seams, and know if Donald had touched his shampoo or soap in the corner of the shower. Ed would become agitated by disruption of his space, and the idea that another person had actually *touched* his things. Each tiny infraction was magnified a thousand times, and it caused actual physical discomfort best described as that feeling you get from sharp nails scratching a chalkboard, creating waves of nausea.

OCD, unchecked and untreated, not only can result in strengthened existing obsessions and compulsions, but also can splinter into a multitude of manifestations. For example, a sufferer who is afraid to enter a room with tile on the floor can suddenly find him- or herself with contamination issues. A student who must repeatedly erase and rewrite her nme on the paper countless times until it is perfect may suddenly be unable to enter a mall with friends without having to exit though the same door. Perhaps a housewife who can't leave her home without checking the lock twenty times is suddenly burdened by intrusive sexual thoughts. There is no logical or predictable path of progression.

Donald's presence triggered the force of Ed's need to have everything in his world in its exact place. At this point, in the summer of 1995, he was still able to venture outside, and he made a trip to the drugstore to buy four sets of bath products for Donald, hoping it would prevent him from using his. But of course, in the ordinary sharing of one's bath and shower, things get moved, touched, and used, and Ed's anxiety escalated. "Everybody saw my behavior as controlling, but anybody who knows who I really am as a person knows that's the last thing I want to do," says Ed. Although the two men remained friends, they did eventually agree to end their shared living arrangement. "That's why I started living in a hell all by myself, because I didn't want to be a burden to anybody," recalls Ed.

By the fall of 1995, Ed spent most of his time alone in the basement as his checking, counting, hoarding, rewinding, and contamination issues began to meld into a conglomeration of rituals that would lead to his eventual solitary confinement. He was not yet fully immersed in what would become his OCD sanctuary. It was on one of those rare days that he decided to invite his friend Donald to eat out at a restaurant about twenty-five miles from Ed's home. Don drove and, after an uneventful, quiet lunch, decided to use the airport rotary on the way home, a detour from the path they had taken to get to the restaurant.

While Don vaguely remembers the incident, Ed recalls with absolute clarity yelling and pleading with him to go another way, or be let out of the car. But Don was in a hurry to get to work and didn't understand the magnitude of Ed's pain. In a state of blinding panic, Ed says he reached for the handle of the door, prepared to jump out of the moving vehicle, but it was too late, the car had already entered the rotary. He became dizzy and nauseated and could barely catch his breath.

Twenty-five miles later, Ed threw the car door open and climbed out of the car onto his driveway, nauseous, exhausted from arguing with Don, and terrified that he had done something that was irreversible and that would have some dire consequence for someone he loved. Ed had to figure out a way to undo the damage.

To passersby who spotted Ed walking backward for the incredible twenty-five mile journey back in time toward the Hyannis rotary, he looked like a crazy person. College boys would taunt him from their car windows and truckers would blow their horns, but he didn't care. He couldn't care. If he didn't do this, he would be consumed with the feeling that something bad was going to happen to someone he loved.

Between episodes of even counting spells throughout the nearly fifty-mile round-trip journey on foot, Ed pushed through the excruciating trek by telling himself to "focus on the big game." These are words he attributes to his role model, Coach Wade from Clemson, and the inspiration he used to keep him going.

Ed departed from his house at seven o'clock at night and didn't return home until shortly before dawn the next morning. He had indeed made the entire trip walking backward, and he'd hustled to make it home before the sun rose. He had started the trip when it was dark and he had to return to his house when it was dark because if the sun had risen, he would have been compelled to do the entire trip over again.

Ed fell into bed exhausted, but he could not fall asleep. He lay there *mentally* rewinding his backward journey, honing in on every misstep. He instinctively knew he had a responsibility to review every time he stepped out of a straight line, every slight stumble, every time his arms and legs weren't in sync—to make things right, so no one would suffer for his mistakes. At one point, his shoelaces became untied, which caused a mental dilemma of epic proportions, because he had to will himself not to tie them for fear that by stopping, he wouldn't complete his task. Now, in the safety of his dad's basement, he had to mentally retie them. Retracing every misstep took over an hour, but he soon released himself from this mental trap and fell asleep.

The entire episode marked a critical new phase in Ed's life where everything became completely clear. His life's purpose was unquestionably to fight the battle against time's progression. It was the only way to stop death. "By keeping everything in reverse, just like watching a VCR movie, reversing the process puts me back ten minutes ago, five minutes ago, which meant I wasn't aging, so no one around me could age and progress toward d-e-a-t-h (spelled out)," says Ed.

# CHAPTER 5

# Something About Michael

⏮

IN 1992, THE SAME YEAR Ed got stuck at the fork in the path on the Clemson University campus, Michael, ironically, got stuck, too. The internationally renowned psychiatrist was sitting in a car outside a Worcester, Massachusetts, medical building paralyzed, physically unable to move. He was drowning in a depression so debilitating that he was unable to get out of the car and walk into the office. It wasn't until the therapist with whom he had an appointment that day came outside and offered to escort him into the building that he was able to move. All of the loss, anger, sadness, and fear from his years in Vietnam had finally caught up with him. Michael was suffering from a sudden onset of posttraumatic stress disorder (PTSD) triggered by a bout of viral en-cephalitis (brain inflammation).

It was during a trip to Thailand and Malaysia, where he was giving talks on OCD, that he contracted the disease. His cognitive function had become severely impaired, and his recovery was fol-lowed by a depression that triggered the PTSD. In a span of one twenty-four-hour period, he went from a gregarious, robust, energetic man to someone who, quite literally, wanted to jump off a bridge.

Michael hadn't experienced the devastating aftereffects of war. He never fell victim to alcoholism and drug addiction upon returning home the way other vets had. "I went to war and came back. I thought everything was fine," he recalls. But in actuality, Michael was far from fine. The memories of friends and innocent Vietnamese civilians killed in a war that, to him, made no sense at all were now at the forefront of his mind. *Why me?* he thought. *Why did I survive?* It was a question with no logical answer, and it consumed him. He remained ambiguous with his colleagues, including the chairman of the Psychiatry Department, who was a friend, about why he was unable to work, telling them only, "I can't do these things right now."

The experiences of a war that happened twenty-four years earlier were only *now* affecting Michael's consciousness, and he would not be allowed to move forward until he dealt with the horrific images that were plaguing his mind. "I didn't even know that I had any traumatic stuff in my head, until this happened," he maintains.

MICHAEL WAS DRAFTED INTO SERVICE just as he finished working on his master's degree in biology at the University of

Massachusetts–Amherst and student deferments had been abolished. But because he was not born in America, and his mother was British, he could have simply avoided the war altogether by acquiring his British passport and stating citizenship. It was an easy out. In fact, he was encouraged by his own father, who had never spoken in detail about his own experience as a soldier in World War II, to take advantage of his English birth and escape the potential horror that awaited him in Southeast Asia. But Michael believed it wrong to live in a country and not perform the duties that being a citizen there entailed. This very patriotic attitude along with an innate affinity for challenge—intellectual *and* physical—made him destined for war.

**BORN IN EDINBURGH, SCOTLAND, MICHAEL** is the oldest son of Andrew Jenike, a distinguished officer of the Polish Army who escaped to England during World War II, and Una, the beautiful, dark-haired model with whom he fell in love after spotting her in a local shop in Ipswich, England. The older Jenike, a mechanical engineering graduate of Warsaw Polytechnic Institute, who later obtained his PhD in structural engineering from the University of London, is today hailed around the world as the "father of mass flow theory."

Michael's grandfather, an employee of the naval academy, a school built for the children and grandchildren of British seafarers, had a home on the grounds overlooking the river Stour, near the village of Holbrook where Michael and his mother lived for a brief time after the war while his father was away in Canada seeking entry into the United States.

When Michael was four years old, he was admonished by his

parents to stay away from an angry bull that roamed the pasture near his home. But the grave danger that awaited him should he ever cross over the white fence separating him from the belligerent creature only served to *entice* the little boy as he walked past the open field with his family on their way to the military parades at the Royal Hospital School in Ipswich.

One day, Michael was playing by this cow pasture all by himself when sheer curiosity compelled the four-year-old to fearlessly set foot over the fence. The bull immediately locked his angry eyes on the tiny intruder, arched its massive back in an aggressive stance, lowered its swaying head, and began pawing at the ground, ready for a good run. Alone, Michael was in serious trouble.

It's difficult to imagine just how hard the heart of a four-year-old beats under pursuit by a two-thousand-pound beast, or how long it takes for a regular rhythm to be restored once its owner is safely perched in the lofty crook of two tree limbs. But there was plenty of time for him to calm down after scrambling to the nearest tree, waiting what seemed an interminable period of time for the bull to lose interest in him and go away.

But while he waited high up in the tree, Michael was preoccupied with another kind of trouble—not the life-threatening kind, but it may have seemed so from a four-year-old's perspective—and that was the scolding surely awaiting him from his mother when he got home.

Michael did get the punishment that was coming to him, but parental discipline couldn't stunt his lifelong predilection for altercation and his inclination to question authority. He welcomed and even *yearned* for challenges, no matter how impossible or potentially fatal they seemed. The words *no, can't* and *don't* to this day seem to trigger an almost primal need within him to search for a way to make the impossible, possible. The greater the challenge, the more emphatic Michael's raison d'être.

Shortly after the bull incident, Michael sailed across the ocean, landing in Niagara Falls with his family, a brief stopover for the Jenikes before his father landed a professorship at the University of Utah in Salt Lake City. The Jenike family, which soon included younger brother Ian, moved many times while living there, until Michael's senior year in high school when they headed east to Winchester, Massachusetts.

The constant shifts between neighborhoods and the changing of schools took a very heavy toll on the very shy Michael. It seemed every school had its own group of bullies barricading the front door, waiting to terrorize the next new kid to enter—and he was *always* that new kid. It was agonizing to be beaten up all the time, but it was even more unbearable for him to watch his younger brother become a target as well.

But Michael recalls the incident where he stopped being a victim. One afternoon, after yet another move, this time simply to a new neighborhood within Salt Lake, he and Ian were approached by a group of older boys. A calm came over him. Suddenly, it no longer mattered to him that the boys who had come around to pick on them were all bigger, and it didn't matter that he was outnumbered; he'd had enough. He took Ian home and came back to fight the boys, alone.

Michael quickly developed a reputation for fearlessness but also for getting in trouble, born of necessity to survive being the new kid at school. Because he was a target for bullies, a very nice boy had suddenly become a behavioral and academic challenge. Michael had been a perennial public school student despite the number of family moves, but now the behavioral problems that ensued led his parents to enroll the fiery eleven-year-old in a more discipline-oriented religious school across town. His parents hoped that the structure would help put him back on the straight and narrow. But Michael's hatred for bullies continued to solidify and now extended to the tyrannical figures that ran his new school.

The headmaster, a strict disciplinarian with a somewhat sadistic bent, arranged grueling boxing matches between his students at lunchtime. Michael remembers having been intentionally paired with a much bigger boy just so the man could watch him take a beating. It was a school where only the strong survived the administration, much less the brutality of the tougher boys. Michael remembers vividly the cruelty displayed by its leadership, and particularly one occasion, when a young Dutch boy whose mother was dying of cancer was struck so hard by the principal that you could see the detail of his fingerprints on the side of the boy's face for the rest of the day. It was a profound and lasting experience for Michael. Going forward, he would be wary of authority and rarely trusting of administrations of *any* sort.

At the age of eleven, Michael was the antithesis of a correspondingly aged Ed Zine, but had the two grown up together at the same time, they surely would have been good friends; Michael, the strong and confident one upon whom Ed could lean after the death of his mother. The kind of brother Michael was to Ian was an indication of the kind of influence he would have been on Ed. An unconditionally compassionate individual whose disdain was limited to those who preyed on people weaker than themselves, he would have dragged Ed out of the house and on to the basketball court, shouldering some of the burden of Ed's troubling life and the secrets that haunted him.

There were no private buses to take Michael to his religious boot camp of a school, so he was left to take the long ride across town on public transportation. His was one of the first stops on the route, and every morning, like clockwork, three stops in, a little old lady would climb aboard the already packed bus. When Michael spotted her coming down the aisle he would pick up his books, rise, and offer his seat, and she would thank him for his kindness. He was quick to inform the woman that he owed his good manners to his mother, "because she was British." The two would often chat between stops as they traveled together down Ninth South Street in Salt Lake City, enjoying their acquaintance. But the following year, Michael's tenure at the private school was over, and it was time to move on to junior high school and start taking the regular school bus.

In junior high school, Michael continued to grow in size, confidence, and personality. And, as is typical of boys during these transitional junior high years, a bigger personality meant bigger disruptions in class. At one point, he was so disruptive in shop class that his teacher grabbed him by the back of the head, took him outside, and parked him face-first in front of a large tree. He told Michael if he liked talking so much, he could spend the rest of the hour talking to the tree. Without missing a beat, the teacher still within earshot, the irascible Michael began a very loud diatribe, "That Mr. Haycock is the worst piece of a shit for a teacher I've ever seen."

Within seconds, the teacher's hand was once again on the back of Michael's neck, pulling him into the administration office. Hand still firmly clasped on his neck, the teacher walked through the principal's door without so much as a knock and screamed, "He was talking to the tree and saying bad things about me!" The ridiculousness of this statement didn't escape Michael, and it was all he could do to stifle the laughter, but the pressure on his neck was intense enough that he couldn't so much as lift his head up to acknowledge his new principal. But as the teacher's grip loosened, he looked up and immediately noticed that sitting behind the desk was the woman for whom he'd given up his seat on the bus every day of the previous school year. Fortunately for him, she recognized him immediately.

If there was one person who could see past his troubled school record, and know with certainty that he was a genuinely sweet, bright boy who deserved consideration and support, it was this woman, whose name, today, escapes him. She dismissed the teacher and asked Michael to sit. He was honest and articulate, especially for someone so young, about his anger toward people who walked around trying to intimidate others and explained to her that his history of fighting (he couldn't get around his records, which contained files of his disruptive behavior) had nothing to do with simply wanting to cause trouble; it was because he simply didn't like bullies. This was not an experience that completely reformed Michael, but for those times when he did get into trouble, it certainly helped to have an advocate.

ANDREW, MICHAEL'S FATHER, TRAVELED A lot while Michael's mother was left alone with the children, trying to get them, and herself, acclimated to America, and the change in scenery with each move. Una was an exceptionally proper and well-mannered woman, and although she certainly had no affinity for American niceties (or lack thereof), she cared very deeply about what others thought of them and was particularly focused on being the sophisticated yet dutiful wife of the prominent professor, keeping up with appearances in academic circles.

A very strong and powerful man, Andrew was the only person Michael ever *really* feared. When he returned home from long business trips, his parents would retreat to their room for private conversations, and while Michael was never really quite sure what was being said about him and his brother, these discussions usually resulted in a whipping.

But despite the rigorous discipline during his youth, in blatant opposition to his mother's desire to cater to public opinion, Michael distanced himself from such feelings of concern; in fact, he couldn't care less what people thought. This attitude, combined with his fearlessness, hatred of bullies, and disregard for authority, created a personality of quiet confidence and internal power that would eventually become a significant part of the unique manner in which he would approach his leadership role in the air force, and in his subsequent medical practice in his treatment of patients. But the most deeply abiding and significant force in Michael's life was his ever-developing compassion for human suffering. For this, he credits his mother.

Una suffered from unrelenting migraine headaches. As a boy, Michael would sit by her side, keeping vigil, until the episode passed, or until she became so desperately ill that she had to go into the hospital for treatment, something that wasn't at all uncommon during his childhood. With his father away much of the time, Michael was the responsible male in the house, and there was little he could do to help his mother but watch, wait, and be available if she needed anything—tea or a glass of water, perhaps—as she suffered through the pain. As a teenager, he would learn to administer injections of Demerol into her arm. Of this responsibility, Michael says, gently, "I didn't mind."

Rounding out his early medical experience were the long summers spent in England with his grandparents. It was a clear precursor to his interest in geriatrics, which was actually his first specialty in medicine. He describes his maternal grandmother as "the most lovable person in the world," and he delighted in the time spent helping her, tending the garden, and going for long walks. Together they cared for his ailing grandfather who'd suffered several heart attacks. While there he would also spend countless hours with his great-aunt Min, to whom he would deliver fish and chips in exchange for some idle banter. Min, who lived to be nearly one hundred years old, would later become the subject of several medical journal editorials authored by Michael on the subject of geriatric medicine.

As much as Michael's time in England would inform his later life, it didn't check his impulsive and even rebellious instincts. He had the heart of a maverick, and at the age of fifteen, after a summer of nurturing his English relatives, he used the money he had accumulated from a paper route to board a jet to Paris rather than return to his family in Utah as planned. His independent spirit was fueled by the growing realization that money spelled freedom for Michael. And with the money he had saved so responsibly, he bought a motorcycle.

In keeping with his self-sufficiency, Michael decided in his senior year of high school that he didn't want to go to college. He felt he had little to gain from the world of academia. He had this heartfelt desire to travel across the country on his motorcycle to get a *real world* education. His *father*, on the other hand, had a very different idea. *His* plan was for Michael to go to MIT, study engineering, and one day take over the business he'd begun as an engineering consultant.

But applying to MIT was the last thing on Michael's mind, so he just didn't. He assumed he would automatically be off the hook when an acceptance letter failed to show up in the mail, but he hadn't counted on his father discovering this deception. By the time Andrew learned of Michael's plan to evade his college applications, MIT's deadline had passed. *Most* deadlines had passed. And with the clock ticking, and just one week left before Tufts University's closing date, Michael was compelled by his father to apply with undesirable results—at least as far as Michael was concerned. He was accepted.

# CHAPTER 6

# Michael's War

⏮

ACADEMICS HELD LITTLE INTEREST FOR Michael, and most of his undergraduate years were spent on the basketball courts, at parties, and pretty much anywhere that was a safe distance from the library and any place that even hinted at academic resource; he often skipped class and trekked to New York City to hang out with friends in Greenwich Village. "I had no plans, and no ambition," says Michael. "I was only there because my father insisted upon it." Organized education was taking the wind out of Michael's sails and dampened his independent spirit. Rarely attending class, but blessed with innate intellectual ability, Michael studied only enough to get him through his scheduled exams. He was suspended on two separate occasions: once for fighting, and once for drinking. By the time he managed to graduate from Tufts in 1967 with an unremarkable C average, the war was raging in Vietnam, and draft numbers were being called with alarming regularity.

So Michael opted for a student deferment and applied to graduate school. Given his less-than-stellar performance at Tufts, and dual suspension record, the odds of success were not in his favor. It was only his God-given ability to test exceptionally well on the Graduate Record Examination that enabled him to receive probationary acceptance to the master's biology program at the University of Massachusetts–Amherst. But by the time he completed his degree, he received his draft notice.

Michael went down right away and underwent his army physical, but having been a scuba diver since high school he thought the navy might be a more interesting option of service for him. However, when representatives of the navy at the naval recruitment center explained that divers spent most of their time doing underwater labor, he reconsidered. *Labor* was not a part of his working vocabulary. So Michael quickly turned his attention to the air force. At the time, the air force was looking for pilots, and it sounded interesting, even exciting—in spite of Michael's fear of heights.

So Michael entered Officer's Training School in San Antonio, Texas, where his scorn for authority and rebellious disposition ran counter to the air force way of life and signaled instant trouble for Michael as he found himself making and breaking his own records for the number of demerits received in one week.

His insubordination clocked him countless miles of punishing marches and a seemingly endless stint as toilet cleaner for his barracks. His time spent bending his tall frame over the white porcelain bowls and kneeling on the cold tile gave him much opportunity to consider war, and he deduced that barracks duties and perfectly folded socks had nothing to do with being a good soldier. By his own estimation, this was all just a ridiculous waste of time. He believed that the air force was brainwashing his fellow officers-in-training into thinking that cleanliness and neatly made beds were integral steps to winning the war, when common sense suggested otherwise.

Common sense—it is one of the most fundamental and important elements that drive Michael's internal compass. Unfortunately, he didn't always have the maturity to express his highly tuned rationale in a way that was appreciated by those around him. In the early days of his Officer and Flight Training Schools, Michael certainly didn't stand on ceremonies. He would laugh out loud in the face of senior officers, screaming at the tops of their lungs, just inches away from his face, and then, to add insult to injury, toss off smart-ass remarks about their bad breath. He once blatantly told another superior that he could "stick the air force up his ass."

An insurgent intellectual whose education and intellect allowed him to reign above his fellow recruits academically, Michael quickly discovered that brightness was far from enough to keep him from getting kicked out of flight school in Enid, Oklahoma. He struggled with proper flight protocol according to military procedure, admitting, "I was much more interested in just cramming up the engines, and speeding around the farms." A maverick was not what the air force needed in the middle of a war that required disciplined fliers and leadership, and clearly Michael lacked the restraint needed to be a good pilot.

"There were certain routes, specific speeds, and a course that needed to be followed," recalls Michael, whose unwillingness to follow the status quo hit critical mass when Lieutenant Colonel Pullins climbed in Michael's assigned plane and took the seat next to him during a practice run. As they flew together, he told Michael he had to do it right, or he was going to get kicked out. This actually instilled a fear in Michael, because it was the first time he was faced with possible expulsion. Reprimands he could deal with; complete failure, not so much. "Before that, I never wanted to be in a position, or job, where I cared enough to stay, but, suddenly, being a good pilot was important to me," says Michael. This was enough to get Michael to "straighten up, and fly right," and by the time he finished his pilot training, he was high enough in the class rankings to pick the specialty school of his choice.

Unlike fighter pilots who were usually stationed in one place and limited to performing short, regimented missions, C-130 transport pilots traveled around the world to different locations, moving men and materials and executing rescue missions. But that's not where the discrepancy stopped. The difference between the two types of pilots was far more grave.

"As a fighter pilot, you're going to random destinations killing people you don't know, and not knowing whether they really deserve to be killed." Michael couldn't justify any of this to himself and even admits that if he found himself in a situation where people might be congregating, he'd probably intentionally misfire. "You don't have a choice but to execute, and that was a whole lot of trouble for me. I wouldn't have shot in the right place if I thought there were people there." But opting to be a transport pilot didn't help to avoid the inevitable, and after finishing C-130 specialty school in Little Rock, Arkansas, Michael headed off to the war.

He was stationed in Taiwan, and when he wasn't on missions,

or partying on his days off with his good friend Stan Mehrhoff, Michael focused on maintaining an extraordinary running routine. He ran twenty miles a day until he was able to run one hundred miles at a fast pace, because he was determined not to get stuck in Vietnam as a prisoner of war. "In survival school, we went to mock POW camps, and I didn't want to have anything to do with that, so I ran, and ran, and ran. I was not going to get captured," he recalls. He figured if his plane went down, he would stand a chance if he could outrun the enemy. In fact, he made a pact with Stan that if one of them *did* get captured, the other would do whatever it took to get his buddy out, even if it meant breaking military protocol and sneaking into Hanoi.

The military experience had managed to smooth the rough edges of a natural-born leader in Michael. "I went from being totally carefree and irresponsible to feeling a strong sense of responsibility for the people in my plane, my crew, and the men I worked with every day." Michael had finally come to a place where he was able to distinguish between the rules and guidelines necessary to ensure the survival of the men he commanded, and those falling outside the boundaries of his own good common sense. He continued to be disruptive, never hesitating to speak up against the norm, but only in a way that *he* felt benefited those he served.

Before the end of the war, Michael would receive countless commendations for his leadership, and performance in Vietnam, including the prestigious Distinguished Flying Cross. The commendation reads:

*"First Lieutenant Michael A. Jenike distinguished himself by extraordinary achievement while participating in aerial flight*

*as a C-130E Pilot for the 345th Tactical Airlift Squadron at*
*Dak To, Republic of Vietnam, on 3 January 1972. On that date,*
*Lieutenant Jenike flew a tactical emergency troop evacuation*
*mission into this hostile short field as the base was being*
*overrun. Despite marginal weather, and intense hostile ground*
*fire, Lieutenant Jenike and his crew successfully landed and*
*evacuated twenty allied troops just as the base of the perimeter*
*was being invaded. The professional competence, aerial skill,*
*and devotion to duty displayed by Lieutenant Jenike reflect*
*great credit upon himself and the United States Air Force.*

Upon reflection, Michael sees nothing extraordinary about
the heroism he demonstrated during the war, saying, "It seems
like heroics, but it really isn't. For most people who've been in a
war, even if they've done heroic things, they don't feel like heroes,
because you're just trained to do it."

From the catbird seat of a cruel war, Michael Jenike would
return home with the rank of captain, with traumas that would
be tucked away for more than twenty years—the result of having
witnessed the atrocities of suffering people and the loss of too
many good men. He came home with a deeply abiding sense of
time and its overwhelming brevity—as well as a goal, a goal not
so far removed from Ed's. Michael likewise wanted to heal the
sick, save lives, and preserve precious moments in time, but his
own aspirations led him to a more practical conclusion: medical
school.

On a trip back to Oklahoma where he'd been stationed before
the war, Michael scheduled an appointment with the dean of the
University of Oklahoma Medical School to find out exactly what
it would take for him to gain admission to their program. It was

made clear to him, in no uncertain terms, that the only way he was ever going to see the inside of medical school was by going back to college for a year, getting straight As, and acing the MCAT. It was a daunting task, but for someone of Michael's intellect and drive, it was not impossible. He just had to regiment himself.

For the next year, while Michael was stationed at Langley Air Force Base in Williamsburg, Virginia, he attended William and Mary College during the day and flew, mostly, at night. His wing commander had a son who wanted to go to medical school, as well, and was very understanding of Michael's goal. A year later, having met *all* requirements, he returned to the University of Oklahoma with an MCAT that placed him in the ninety-ninth percentile, which indicates the highest achievement on a standardized test.

MICHAEL DISCOVERED THAT MOST OF his classmates had lived lives that hadn't predisposed them to real human tragedy the way he had. His perspective, he felt, was noticeably different. In Vietnam, Michael was in a place where people didn't simply use death as a metaphor. He was quite serious about his studies, but he couldn't sympathize with the perfunctory concerns about test results. So, although he paid attention in class and took his studies seriously, when it came time to decide between studying an extra hour or shooting hoops, it didn't take long for him to reach for his basketball. He certainly could never be accused of studying *too* hard, and he simply allowed his natural abilities to propel him straight to the head of the class.

Michael entered medical school intent on becoming a surgeon. In fact, when he left the service, he already had the rational mentality of a surgeon, which was, "If there's a problem, let's fix it." In part, this was a natural extension of his pragmatic personality, but it was also reinforced by his training as a pilot and the need to make quick, lifesaving decisions. Despite his sensibility, however, he couldn't separate himself from his innate compassion, and a desire for quick solutions didn't supersede his personal interest in patients' welfare.

On one occasion during his medical school tenure, Michael and a fellow student were given the assignment to interview a sick patient who also happened to be a prison inmate. While his classmate, who ultimately became a heart surgeon, focused on asking pointed questions about the man's symptoms, Michael found himself more interested in asking him about why he was in prison in the first place, which actually frustrated the future surgeon and caused verbal conflict between the two *at* the interview as the other student chided him in front of the patient, deeming these questions about the inmate's criminal past immaterial. But Michael had developed an interest in diseases of the mind and subconscious motivation, and he began gravitating toward psychiatry. He found great role models in men like Dr. Ronald Krug, Dr. Gordon Deckert—chairman of the psychiatry department and a nationally respected lecturer—and Dr. John Rush, an international expert on depression and cognitive therapy, among many of the other great teachers who congregated at Oklahoma, and pursued a psychiatry elective.

Michael's concern for his patients' emotional, and physical, welfare extended beyond the long hours he spent at the hospital in training. So much so, in fact, that in his third year, even after spending long hours covering his regular duties at the hospital, he would make home visits, driving to the homes of terminally ill lung cancer patients to drain the fluid from their lungs. "I hated to see people end their lives in hospitals when their families wanted them to die at home in comfort," says Michael.

While on rotation at the local VA hospital, Michael was assigned to a patient who suffered from horrendous stomach pain, which was dismissed by his physician as psychosomatic. The man, undaunted, planned to go to another hospital for a second opinion, and he requested his medical records from the administration. The hospital staff, citing protocol, said they could not officially release his medical records for several weeks. So Michael, always the renegade, took it upon himself to walk into the Medical Records Department, secretly extract the patient's records and X-rays, and deliver them into the hands of the patient, who waited outside in his car. The man's consultation revealed that the pain from which he was suffering was not in his head at all. He had a metastatic melanoma—skin cancer—that spread to his internal organs.

Michael's action was not intended to be taken as an act of public defiance—he simply wanted the patient to be able to have the consult that he deserved, which Michael felt was well within his rights. The bureaucratic delays made no sense at all and would have only served to cause his patient greater suffering. "In the military, there are rules that keep you from getting shot down," says Michael. "But if there's someone who needs to be rescued, you have to take the risk and do whatever you have to do to get them out."

IN 1978, MICHAEL GRADUATED FROM the University of Oklahoma Medical School at the top of his class. He received, by unanimous vote, the school's first "Solomon Papper Humane Scholar Award." Following his graduation from medical school, he accepted a psychiatric residency at the prestigious Massachusetts General Hospital in Boston and a clinical fellowship at Harvard University Medical School. It was here that he encountered a more sophisticated, educated type of bully.

During his first few months of residency, Michael had a standard rotation in the Acute Psychiatric Care Unit of the Emergency Room. In the first month, he encountered a surgeon who was yelling, relentlessly, at one of the psychiatric residents on duty for something that Michael felt was pointless. The young guy was terrified. So the strong ex-pilot took matters into his own hands, literally. He grabbed the surgeon, introduced his back to the wall, and let him know in no uncertain terms that he should never, ever come back into the unit and scream at another resident like that again.

The second Michael released the stunned surgeon, he realized his residency was all but certainly finished. Within minutes after walking away, he heard his name being paged over the hospital loudspeaker to come to the office of the chief of psychiatry, Dr. Tom Hackett. It was a flashback to his junior high school days, when that call was for him to come to the principal's office, but he was prepared to live with the consequences of his actions, because he felt that intervening was the right thing to do. After explaining what had happened, Michael recalls that Dr. Hackett said, "'Good job,' and told me to get back to work."

In his new Ivy League environment, Michael continued to challenge the traditions and rules that didn't make sense to him. He wasn't looking for a fight, and he didn't need the attention or the accolades; he just followed his standard approach to life.

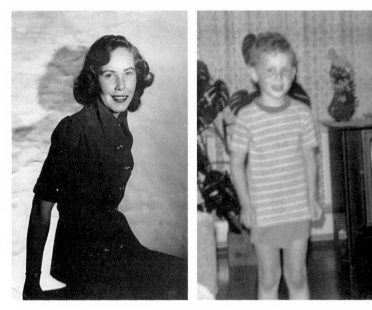

Rita Grace Zine, Ed's mom.          Ed Zine, around age four.

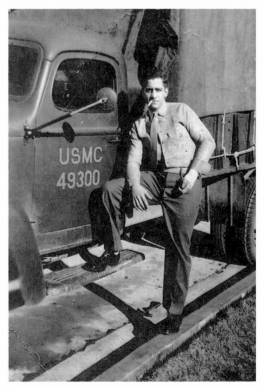

Bob Zine, Ed's dad.

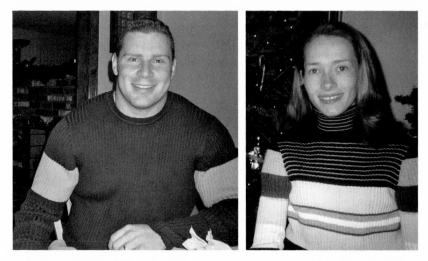

Ed.

Mayada.

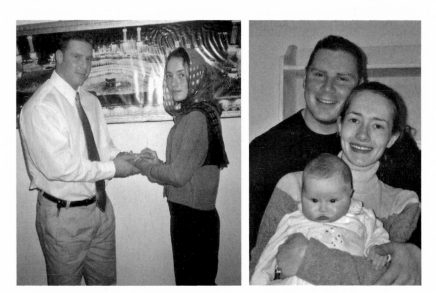

Ed and Mayada on their wedding day.

Ed, Mayada, and Alexandria.

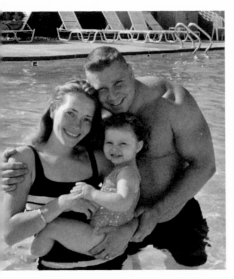

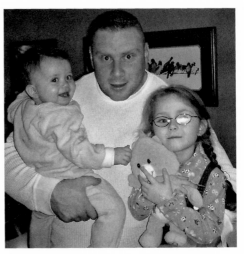

Mayada, Alexandria, and Ed in 2002.          Ed with Isabella and Alexandria in 2006.

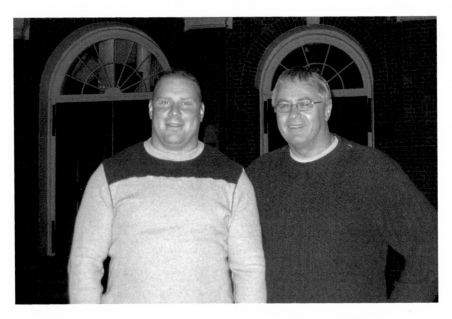

Ed and Michael in 2008.

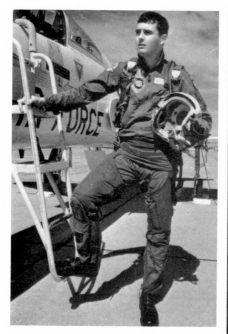

Lieutenant Michael Jenike, 1970.

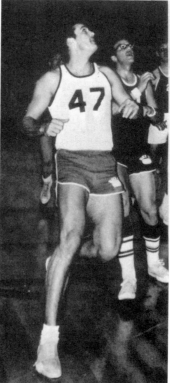

Michael, 1970.

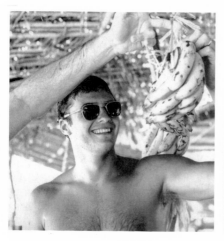

Michael on an island near Thailand.

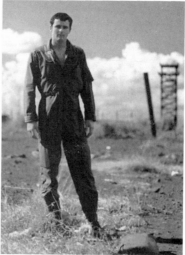

Michael at the Song Be Perimeter,
Vietnam.

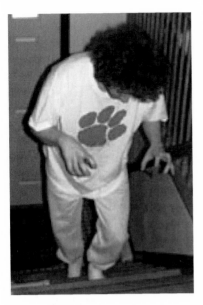

Ed climbing the steps from the basement to the living room. Picture taken by Dr. Michael Jenike, May 1998.

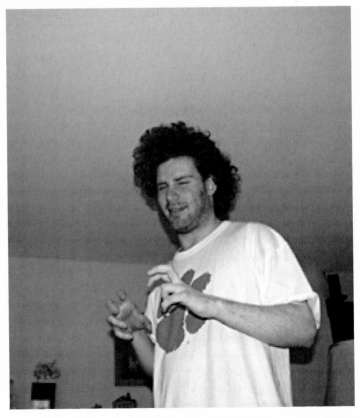

Picture of Ed taken by Dr. Michael Jenike in Ed's home, May 1998.

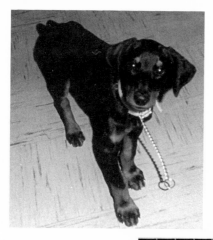

Zeus, 1993.

Alexandria's sonogram.
She's looking right at Ed.

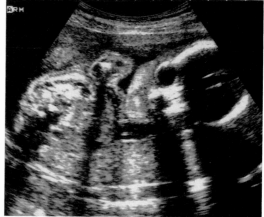

Ed and Don Post.

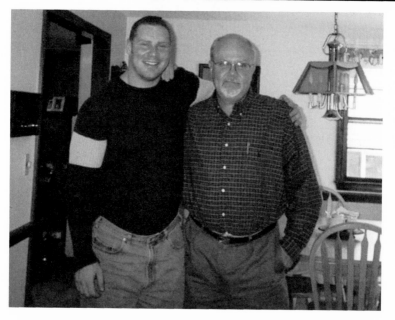

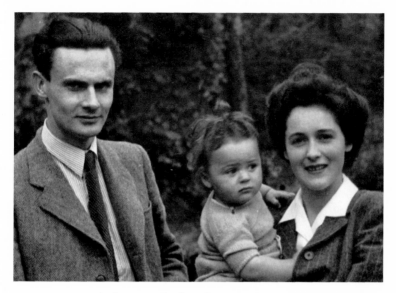

Andrew, Michael, and Una Jenike, 1946.

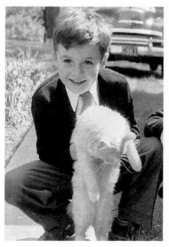

Michael and friend.

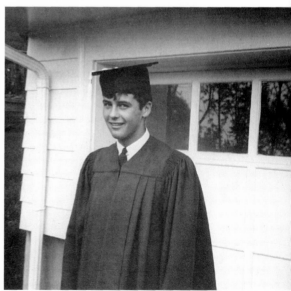

Michael at his high school graduation, 1963.

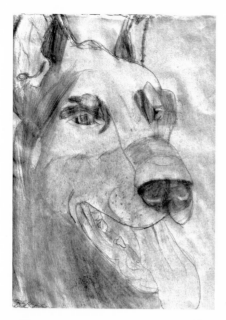

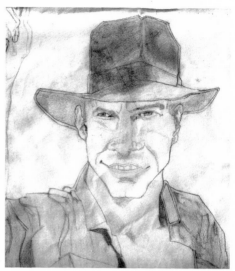

Ed's animation art.

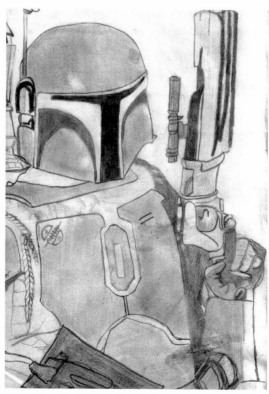

"Mike has a strong sense of right and wrong, and if he finds 'wrong,' he's going to do something about it," says Dr. Krug. "You don't want to cross him in a way that is meant to take advantage of someone, particularly if somebody is being nasty for the sake of being nasty, because he doesn't mind stepping in if it's the right thing to do."

**THE SAME MONTH MICHAEL GRADUATED** from medical school, the introductory note of a report published in the *American Journal of Psychiatry* gave a brief commentary on the state of psychiatric house calls during that time, noting that psychiatrists rarely ever made house calls and participated in that "special world on the individual's private territory." "Michael immediately broke from this norm," recalls Dr. Krug, "recognizing the importance of house calls as a tool to help patients in severe distress who might not otherwise get help."

There were doctors who criticized him for making house calls, telling him that he got overinvolved with his patients. But, as was Michael's wont, he just kept on doing it. One particular case involved a young homeless kid in his twenties who suffered from alcoholism. "He would come into the Emergency Room—filthy, nasty, dirty—and I would spend time with him," says Michael. "We'd eat breakfast, lunch, and dinner, and by dinnertime he'd actually start to make sense." But though he was criticized for befriending and mentoring the young man, extending the relationship beyond the typical boundaries of the doctor-patient relationship, Michael believed this was the kind of attention that would penetrate. The young man needed a friend and an advocate.

Eventually, the young man, who was a very talented musician, sobered up and managed to get off the streets. Many of Michael's colleagues at Mass General failed to appreciate Michael's ability to draw his own lines and innately comprehend when a situation was in fact becoming *too* personal. But Michael's approach wasn't anarchic in any sense. He knew the lengths to which he could go with a patient without the situation becoming inappropriate. "He'll stick out his hand, but he doesn't rescue anybody," notes Dr. Krug. "If a person starts to lean too heavily on Mike, he'll tell them to get off his back."

So, just like the renegade doctors on prime-time medical dramas who will perform risky procedures on a newborn or overstep their boundaries for the good of an elderly patient, Michael was scrutinized and had his practices impugned by those above him. And since he often chose to speak up against the prevailing system, he would not be assigned as much time with trainees as some of his counterparts. But it didn't matter, because Michael was an extraordinarily effective clinician and researcher. In time, his instinctual reactions, impulsivity, and extra efforts with patients would earn the respect of his dubious colleagues when his methods would lead to unprecedented success in the area of obsessive-compulsive disorder. He would establish the first privately funded residential patient facility for OCD in the country, and he would later become the direct recipient of the largest single donation ever received by any department in the entire history of Massachusetts General Hospital.

MICHAEL JENIKE IS A KIND and gentle man, the rock that his patients, friends, and family lean on for a touch of reassurance as they try to find their own inner strength. But in 1992 it was

Michael who was dealing with painful bouts of despondency and helplessness—and he knew that he needed the same kind of help his patients typically needed so he could deal with the trauma and achieve progress.

That year, while in the care of a therapist and while under hypnosis, Michael visited the Vietnam Veterans Memorial in Washington, D.C., looking for the names of friends who had been lost in the war. What he found was his own name written across that wall. It had been twenty years since his return from the war, and he was suddenly overcome by an overwhelming guilt that came from living while friends had been lost. He owed it to those young friends and soldiers, who never got a chance to fulfill vast amounts of potential, to continue serving a population of under-served patients, to a point where he could recognize and fulfill the slim potential for healing in an otherwise hopeless patient named Ed Zine.

# CHAPTER 7

# Trapped in the Basement

◀◀

HUNDREDS OF SMALL BLACK ANTS were gnawing at the
flesh of Ed's leg. They'd come in search of food that had fall-
en from his mouth. The line stretched all the way from his foot
to his knee as he watched, paralyzed, carefully weighing the cost
of their painful bites against the thousands of torturous touching
and retouching rituals he would have to perform if he moved.

In the spring of 1996, Ed spent the majority of his days and
nights sitting on the end of his bed in front of the television. It
became his sofa, his toilet, and his kitchen table. His efforts at
personal hygiene had nearly ground to a halt. His daily activities
included an occasional trip down the hall to make a phone call,
and a once-a-day walk to the basement door leading outside to

the driveway where his family would drop off carefully prepared meals in packets of even numbers of Ziploc bags.

OCD is a demanding mistress—unchecked and untreated, it mushrooms. As its victims find clever ways to assuage the anxiety of their obsessions through ritualistic behavior, relief from the anxiety comes, but it is fleeting. OCD can splinter off into new manifestations—counting and checking can often lead to hand-washing or hoarding rituals—and seemingly small obsessions can grow exponentially. In the early stages, the intensity of Ed's OCD came in waves, but now it was an unrelenting force every second of every day.

Ed's OCD was as much about the smallest movements of his body as it was about the big ones. He even monitored the movements of his tongue to make sure it didn't touch his lips and thus possibly set off a series of multiple hours' worth of counting and retouching rituals to relieve the anxiety of that first accidental touch. Eating his food was a test of endurance as he struggled to find ways to slide it down his throat, unable to chew, lest his top set of teeth touch his bottom set.

*Pick up plastic fork without allowing fingers to touch each other, only plastic of fork. Put plastic fork into Ziploc bag, carefully, making sure not to touch sides of bag with fork. If you do, start all over again. Twirl fork around to wrap pasta around end of fork. Do this until there are no hanging strands of pasta so that when you gently pull fork out of bag, no food will touch sides of plastic. If it does, start all over again. Lift fork up at an angle, away from face, and slowly let pasta slide off fork toward open mouth. Shake fork a little, if necessary,*

*and let food fall into mouth. If a strand of pasta touches face,
lip, or chin, and does not go into mouth, gently try to grab
strand with thumb and index finger of other hand, letting
fingers touch only pasta, not each other. If fingers touch each
other, reverse entire process and start over. Make sure fingers
do not touch face or lips. If they do, start touching and
counting rituals—touch skin on face with thumb and then
index finger . . . right, left, right, left, right, left . . . repeatedly
until comfortable . . . multiples of even numbers, sometimes
up to magic number of 16,384. Lift up piece of pasta, and let
fall into mouth without causing any more damage. When food
is in mouth, push in farther by a series of back and forth
movements with fork. Pay close attention to exactly how far
fork can go without going past the point of no return, and
touching mouth on inside. If it does, reverse process and start
all over again. Swallow. Next bite.*

At this point, perhaps unsurprisingly, showering and brushing his teeth had also become an extreme process of mental calculations for the placement of fingers, the touch of bristles, the
direction of movements, and the memory of each drop of water.

*Hold toothbrush in hand without letting fingers touch,
carefully, put in mouth, go in and touch teeth and gums
trying to go back same way, doing exact same stroke back
and forth, touching upper gum, and feeling a bristle, then
trying to reverse it. Keep tongue from touching lips. If bristle
flairs up underneath gum during stroke, replicate movements
backward, while doing normal brushing back and forth, back*

*and forth, in multiples of even numbers. If any movements are done incorrectly, or feel uncomfortable, reverse them, rewind entire process. Start again.*

Each drop of water that hit Ed's skin felt like the jab of a needle, but he obviously couldn't make the water go back into the showerhead, so he devised a mental compromise. He would create mental images of the water returning from his body to the showerhead, and the soap disappearing from his body back into the bar, until he could feel the event had never happened. He would then spend seven to ten hours rewinding his "mental videotape" of the shower, trying to remember *exactly* where he was standing with each scrub, along with the exact placement of his arms, hands, head, and face. By the time Michael made his first visit to Ed in May of 1996, he had stopped showering and brushing his teeth altogether. The mental and physical exhaustion by that point had trumped the desire for cleanliness.

After going months without a shower, Ed couldn't stand the smell of his own body. He had begun to develop bedsores on his hips and raw skin under his arms where they constantly brushed against his ribs. Looking for relief from the stench, in desperation he picked up a bottle of ammonia-based glass cleaner, lifted his arm, and sprayed it. The pain was excruciating—his skin was on fire—but it didn't stop there. His OCD required him to lower his arm and do a touching ritual of rubbing his arm against the rib around his chest more than a hundred times in order to get the relief he needed to "erase" the event, and thus the *anxiety* that the cleaning process caused, which was as torturous as the physical pain. Alone in his basement, he told himself over and over,

"Stop being a punk!," military-drill-sergeant style, in order to push through the painful event.

Trapped in the basement, there was little distinction between day and night. The television was Ed's daytime companion by which he set the clock of his life, and the night-light by which he slept. He tried to find comfort in movies, avoided the news, and watched a lot of golf—a game he'd never previously enjoyed—to get an emotional lift. Looking at the lush greens on beautiful sunlit days was the closest feeling he could get to being outdoors. But no matter what Ed watched, he would always rewind the programs back and forth in his head, sounding out the words and sentences in reverse in order to hold back the progression of time.

When he got tired, he would use his hands, which he now kept frozen in a clawlike position, fingers spread apart to avoid touching one another, to push himself back on the bed.

*First right hand down, push, then left hand down, push, never let fingers touch one another. Lift right cheek up, and back, push, left cheek up, and back, push. Reverse process a few times, always in multiples, making sure backs of thighs don't catch end of bed. Repeat process back and forth several times until it feels right, sliding all the way back onto middle part of bed. Body locked into position, hands locked into place, fingers spread, lay back, arms resting on elbows, hands up in air, do several times, back and forth, back and forth, until body "feels" perfectly placed. Stop. Don't move. Close eyes. Sleep.*

At the peak of his illness, nights where Ed could simply sink back, curl into a fetal position, and drift off to sleep the way most people might were nonexistent. There were times when he was so busy with his mental calculations and rewinds that he couldn't stop to lie down, and he would fall asleep sitting upright on the end of his bed. Even sleep itself was never comfortable, because in his dreams he would picture the events of the day, the movies and shows he watched, and have to rewind his mental videotape, erasing events from his time continuum, demonstrating the way even his subconscious fell victim to the OCD.

THE HOUSE ABOVE WAS SILENT as Ed struggled with the weight of keeping time in its place so he could keep his family alive and well. By this point, Ed's father was remarried and living elsewhere, immersed in a new life that had little to do with Ed. Deena had a husband and two small children, and Tom was married. Ed's sister Tami, single with two children, assumed primary responsibility for Ed's well-being, and she was the one he counted on the most.

Getting Tami on the phone was a half-day event for Ed. The phone sat on a shelf at the end of a long corridor outside Ed's bedroom in the basement, and simply reaching it required thousands of movements.

*Get up from bed by rocking back and forth, balancing carefully to gain enough momentum to propel body forward into standing position without using hands to push off, and without getting too much momentum that might cause a collision with television opposite bed. Once up, if it doesn't "feel" right, reverse process, and start again. If a sound occurs outside, reverse entire process, and start again. Step*

*carefully . . . right, left, right, left, step over threshold, step
left, right, left, right, left, take right foot, step over another
threshold, stretch legs to point of a near split, but do it and
be careful not to slip, because socks have been on feet for
months and are slimy from filth attached to thinning bottoms.
Steady on right leg—this is hard because leg muscles have
deteriorated from weight loss, and lack of movement so be
careful—hold left leg up, and step out to left to make turn
in hallway. Bring right foot over, take one small step and,
throughout entire process take mental and physical snapshots
of placement of each foot, so it can be exacted on way back
from phone. Simultaneously, count number of times arms
move and take note of where they are at each juncture of
foot placement. Make sure that foot and arm movements are
in exact sequence of even numbers of multiples. Rock back
and forth between each step, closing eyes, counting numbers
while identifying placement of all body parts within memory,
and make sure to stop rocking on an even number. If something goes wrong, rewind all the way back to the beginning,
and start all over, again. Make sure everything in room
remains the same going, and coming. If Tommy stops by,
unexpectedly, and has entered house upstairs, begin entire
rewind from that point, and start all over, again. If you hear
something on television while exiting bedroom, stop, memorize what is being said, replay it backward in mind until
comfortable.*

There were days that a trip to the phone could take up to ten
hours, and then picking up the receiver and *dialing* presented a
completely new set of rituals.

*Pick up, put down, pick up, put down. Do until comfortable, then dial "0" to get operator. Hang up. Do it again. When you repeat to the point of comfort, tell operator you're sick. Zone out for a minute while you replay the conversation in your head. Tell her number you're trying to reach, replay it in your head, say again to get to an even number, replay it in your head. Tell her you will have to call same number several times in even numbers of multiples before you will finally be okay to talk to person on other end of line. Hope she understands and helps. If Tami is not home, worry about whether or not she's all right. Repeat process until you reach her. When Tami still doesn't answer, don't go back to room because it takes too long. Wait. Freeze in place. Replay conversations with operator and numbers all over in head. Think back to when you last knew for sure that Tami was okay. Stay there for a minute. Replay visual of seeing Tami happy and smiling. Think about Star Wars. Freeze. Run back through videotape, scanning, searching. Is everything perfect? Did you fail to protect her? Did she D-I-E (spelled)? Stay in place, by the phone, rock back and forth replaying the moments of your life, all the way back to the last time you saw Tami over and over again.*

**IT WAS SATURDAY MORNING, AND** Tami's phone started ringing early. She knew it was her brother. He'd tried calling her the night before while she was out, and now he was worried. She wanted to just pick up the phone, tell him everything was fine, and that she'd call him later, but she couldn't because there was no such thing as a quick conversation with Ed. If she picked up the phone, she'd get stuck talking to him for hours because he needed unending reassurance that she and the kids were OK.

Ed's continued need for reassurance, the demand for it, is a classic piece of the obsessive-compulsive disorder puzzle, but the problem is that reassurance doesn't really *reassure* someone with OCD—it only serves to create a greater demand for more reassurance.

If you have a family member with OCD, you almost inevitably get pulled into the vortex of its demands and become a peripheral victim of the disorder. "When one person tries to help the person with OCD, it takes a part of their life, too," says Ed. "It's like a vampire sucking the life out of them. If I'm calling you because I'm sick, I'm calling you for solace, or comfort, reassurance. If you're healing me, it's like a baton has been passed, and you've given part of your strength to help me get better."

Whether it's the afflicted person's need for constant reassurance, or a string of demands, families and friends suffer behavior that is controlling, demanding, and even rude, but it's important to isolate the sufferer from his behaviors, which are simply uncontrollable.

On this day, Tami had to choose between speaking with Ed and attending to her children, who were at home and in need of attention at that particular moment. But she knew the more Ed called without a response, the more distressed he would become, and the more calls he would make. Plus she remembered a recent time she wasn't available, when a lightbulb blew out in Ed's room, which left him standing in one spot, rocking back and forth for hours, unable to move, until a typical series of rituals allowed him to unlock himself. But it took sixteen hours to replace the bulb from the time it blew. Tami didn't want that to happen to Ed again.

"Eddie's pain became my pain," remembers Tami. "I would try to find certain words or phrases that would put him in a calm state and repeat them over and over. I couldn't think of him standing in one place, stuck for hours." For the most part, Tami ignored the criticism of her family and friends and tried to balance her efforts with Ed. Tami was the perfect example of a loved one victimized by OCD. She couldn't stand to see her brother suffer, even if she was, in fact, unwittingly exacerbating his condition.

"I had to try and release Eddie so he could feel comfortable simply hanging up the phone at night," says Tami, but "releasing" meant offering reassurances and then allowing him the time he needed to repeat all of the words he spoke multiple times.

OCD took its toll on Deena, the sister closest in age to Ed, as well. She was a newlywed, married right after Ed got out of high school, and now she had two young daughters. Looking at the wedding pictures, which include Ed, there is no indication of the trouble brewing below the surface. Her husband, David, owner of a local fish market, says, "It was like someone turned on a switch. Ed was such a nice, quiet kid who never got into any kind of trouble. There was just no way you could have guessed that he would spiral so far down like that." He also says that Ed's OCD put an enormous amount of pressure on their marriage.

After long hours of running the market, David just wanted to come home, relax, and spend time with his family, but Deena would often be busy cooking up a special order of spaghetti that she would stuff into plastic bags and take to her brother. "The minute I walked through the door, she'd leave to go take care of Eddie, and be gone anywhere from thirty minutes to a couple of hours while I watched the girls, and we'd fight about it," remembers David. To relieve the stress on David, Deena started taking the girls with her.

"The calls were constant, sometimes as many as eight times in a row," she says. It was difficult for the new mother, who was trying to juggle naps for a toddler and new baby. "Sometimes," she remembers, "I would argue with Ed on the phone, and say, 'You have to stop, because David is going to get mad.'"

Ed recalls the tension between Deena and David in the early years of their marriage, and he confirms it would often spill over into his phone conversations with Deena, the anxiety on both ends of the line palpable. He beat himself up for what his OCD was doing because, deep down, he didn't want to bother anyone. The irony was that the anxiety he was causing his sister actually made his own worse. OCD is a breeding ground for these sorts of vicious cycles—the disease, left untreated, constantly feeding on itself.

But despite her domestic difficulties, Deena, ultimately acquiescing to Ed's demands, would call him, let the phone ring four times, and hang up to let him know she was coming. When she arrived, she would leave the girls in their car seats and make her way down the concrete steps to the side door of the basement. The door would be cracked open about six inches, and Ed would be standing behind it. Through the opening, she would pass the packets of warm pasta and two bottles of Gatorade.

"Deena would be torn between the kids in the car, and Ed," David remembers Deena telling him. "Then, by the time she came home, the girls would be sound asleep (in their car seats), and I would have no time with them." The stress between the couple mounted as Deena, who is the spitting image of her mother, not only was attempting to help her brother, but also was still trying to come to grips with her own unresolved issues surrounding her mother's death. According to David, "No one in the family has ever really grieved over the loss of their mother." Only recently, he admits, has Deena begun to open up and really start to talk about it.

Tom Zine, one of the youngest members of the local police department, had always been the responsible older brother, and watched over his mother in the days she struggled with her ailing health, when his father was conspicuously aloof. In high school, he even went to work at the local hospital to bring home some extra money to put in her pocket. But after she died, he left home and joined the army, so he wasn't around in those early difficult days of Ed's mourning, and he carried around some guilt for what had become of Ed. But when he returned from the service, he tried to do what he could to help his kid brother. He would drive by the house during his lunch breaks so he could pick up the mail and check on Ed. Tom also would perform a series of rituals to satisfy the demands of Ed's OCD. Before arriving, like Deena, he would call Ed and let the phone ring four times to announce the time of his arrival. This allowed Ed to get into "waiting position." Depending on how early the warning call came in, he would stand two, three, or four hours in one place waiting for someone to arrive. He would stand and stare into space, zoning out until he heard the clicks of the dead bolt between the upstairs and the basement, which would have to be turned an even number of times. On the fourth click, with Ed in what he calls his "perfection position," Tom could come in. When he left the house, he would have to reverse the process completely, opening and closing the door an even number of times, until Ed felt okay that Tom had erased his own entry into the house, and no time had passed.

**TO THE MEN SITTING IN** the unmarked van across the street, the unusual way that Tom entered the house looked highly suspicious. A uniformed cop doing what appeared to be some strange, secret, coded entrance was significant because Ed's house was under surveillance by the Cape Cod Drug Task Force, which included members of the national Drug Enforcement Agency, the state and local police, and the sheriff's department.

If someone had told Tom that Ed was under surveillance by the Drug Task Force he would have thought it was a sick joke; there was absolutely no way his brother could mastermind a drug-trafficking operation when he could barely get up from the end of his bed. But for the members of the task force sitting outside watching the house, it was no laughing matter. And now Tom was under suspicion, too.

Only a handful of people knew that Ed was living back at home during this time. "Eddie disappeared right in front of our noses," says his friend Phil. "Most of us thought he was back at Clemson doing his thing. Nobody knew he was right down the street, as sick as he was." But for one person who did know that Ed was trapped in his basement, mentally ill, it was a secret worth keeping because it meant an opportunity to make money. This was Ed's high school friend "Ken," who made money on the side delivering drugs sent up from a dealer in Florida. For $500 a pop, he would pick up packages mailed to Cape Cod and deliver them to the buyer.

Knowing that Ed couldn't go upstairs, Ken decided to have

the illicit packages sent via UPS to a fictitious name at Ed's address. He says he wasn't worried about putting Ed in any kind of legal jeopardy because "Eddie didn't know anything about it, and we knew if something went down, they couldn't bust him because he was a mental patient."

On the days of the week that shipments were scheduled to arrive, Ken would make a hot batch of fresh pasta and deliver it to Ed in two plastic bags—an even number. He would call Ed and let the phone ring four times to let him know he was on his way, drive over to the house, pull into the driveway, walk down the steps, pass the packages of food through the door, and sit down and talk to Ed through the opening. They would talk about their friends away at college, women, sports, and movies they'd seen on television.

Having company was a bonus for Ed, and it meant fewer days that he had to burden his family with the responsibility of his meals. For a few months, everything went on without a hitch— but then a confidential informant in Florida dropped a dime.

On the day the eventual last shipment of drugs was scheduled to arrive, Tom was approached at the station by a senior detective who asked him if he wanted to ride along on a drug raid that day. It was pretty heady stuff for a young cop, but Tom was, of course, all in. He was told to stick around the station rather than head out to the streets and, within an hour, he was escorted into the police chief's office. Behind closed doors, Tom was told that $20,000 in street value worth of marijuana had been picked up on its way to being delivered to the house where Ed lived.

Tom understandably thought there had been some mistake. Of course Ed was incapable of being involved in a drug deal, but the only way he could vouch for Ed's innocence was to publicly acknowledge his condition, which he had, to this point, tried so hard to conceal. (The exception was the limited disclosure that was needed when the family had Ed committed in 1995 to Pembroke Hospital, believing he was suicidal.) Tom's job was on the line, and he knew it. What's more, he knew Ed was sitting alone in the basement sitting at the end of his bed, performing his rituals—and he knew that a task force busting through the door could have devastating repercussions to Ed's psyche.

Earlier in the day, the dealer who shipped the drugs from Florida arrived in Cape Cod, waiting just a couple miles down the road from Ed's house. He'd spent two hours driving up and down Route 28, scanning the main thoroughfare that the UPS truck would have to use before turning into Ed's neighborhood. He was on the lookout for the truck, just to make sure it safely arrived at its destination, and watched as the cops pulled the UPS truck over and searched it down. "He called me," says Ken, "and said 'Don't pick up the package, they're coming.'"

At the station, Tom tried to explain Ed's mental illness to the chief, but he was taken to another room and restricted from using the phone until his story checked out and he was finally allowed to speak with the commander of the Drug Task Force. It was a humiliating experience for a good cop like Tom who was trying to fly under the radar while he earned his stripes on the force.

"I was standing in front of everybody, making this big pitch for my brother," he recalls. "I was pleading for them to believe me." It was a desperate situation, because, living in a small town, everybody knows everybody else. Tom knew people would talk, but at this very moment, he had to help his brother and worry about dealing with the social and possibly *professional* repercussions later.

Tom's story was finally verified by the supervisor and the cops who had gone out to the house when Ed had been committed the previous year, and the raid was called off. But investigators would still need to go in and talk to Ed.

Tom was given the latitude to manage the scene at the house, and he directed the team around to the front of the house while he entered through the basement. They wanted Ed to make a phone call to try and pinpoint Ken's location. Ed was in a panic when Tom came to the door and suggested that he would have to come in to the basement and that a few of his fellow officers would have to come in to the house and talk to him through the upstairs door. His heart rate sped up, and he started to sweat profusely. All he could think about was what they might touch or, worse, move. It was like the Pembroke incident all over again. As thin and frail as he was, Ed remembers thinking that he would have to "bull-rush" them before allowing anyone to touch his things.

But Ed says Tom ran "great interference," and when the task force members saw the condition he was in, and how sick he really was, they took extra care to respect his space. Sitting on the steps outside the inside door leading to the basement, the officers told Ed what Ken had done—that he had been betrayed. Ken may not have been his closest friend, but he was the one friend who remained in town while everyone else was at college, or too busy with their lives to stay in touch. And it's not like Ed wanted to pick up the phone and reveal his condition to everyone he knew. So, with Ken as his sole contact outside the family, Ed says, "I didn't want to believe that Ken had anything to do with it, because that would have devastated me. I had to honor all the good things that he'd done for me. That's all I knew." Eventually, Ed had no choice but to make the call to Ken as the police asked, but, still conflicted about his involvement, he refused to press him for information. Later, members of the task force arrested him across the street from his house in Cape Cod.

Even after Ed was presented the documented proof of Ken's crime, it was difficult for him to reconcile the situation because Ken had seemingly been a good friend for a long time—someone who brought him food and took the time to sit on the steps while the two shared memories from happier times. Despite the fact that Ken clearly deserved the punishment he received, Ed missed him, as his life became more lonely, and isolated.

# CHAPTER 8

# The Betrayal

⏮

THE ZINE FAMILY FIRST BECAME aware of a possible link between Ed's symptoms and OCD in the spring of 1995, when Tami shared his story with a therapist friend who surmised he might have the disorder and agreed to see Ed in her office. Ed remembers meeting with her one time, but it was at a time when his OCD was in a waning phase, and he wasn't comfortable with counseling, so he never returned for a second visit.

But in December, Ed experienced another major setback when his dog, Zeus, passed away. Zeus provided an unconditional love that Ed felt he had been missing since the death of his mother, and now, once again, he felt the unbearable pangs of guilt over what he felt was his failure to save both his mother and Zeus. The deaths, to Ed, were not mutually exclusive.

As Christmas drew nearer, Ed began to reach out to family members by phone, or when they stopped in, he asked them to come back and check on him. His self-isolation had, not surprisingly, resulted in loneliness and, consequently, depression; but Tom, now home from the service, felt there was something even more ominous in his appeal. Both he and Tami, who struggled to find time for Ed in her own busy schedule as a single mother raising two children, feared that with the loss of Zeus on the thirteenth anniversary of their mother's death, Ed might be suicidal.

"I called the local mental health clinic," says Tom, "and I talked to a counselor who listened to the story, and he suggested that Ed might be schizophrenic, and possibly a danger to himself. He suggested to me that Ed be 'pink slipped.'" Pink slipped is a term often used by medical and police personnel for being involuntarily committed to a psychiatric hospital.

Although Tom was heartbroken at the thought, he knew he had to talk with the rest of his family and do what was in Ed's best interest. To the Zine family, this meant protecting him from himself and having him committed. The family was simply out of answers.

Tom went to his shift supervisor and told him that Ed was going to be pink slipped, and, on the day of the intervention, Tom was given all the police backup he felt he needed to get Ed to the hospital. But he was afraid of the emotional trauma he would inflict on Ed upon breaching his living quarters, and, logistically, the resistance he would encounter on trying to get him out of the house. "The thought of moving anything down there even a quarter of an inch was devastating, so I couldn't imagine how difficult it was going to be to get him out of the basement," says Tom.

Despite the good intentions, the Zines' approach actually demonstrated how ill educated they were about OCD. But the Zines are not unique. In many cases, Michael Jenike points out, general psychiatric units are not prepared to deal effectively with OCD, and forced admission can make the situation worse. However, it was particularly ironic in Ed's case that his family feared he would take his own life; Ed's obsession was all about *preventing* death, not fostering it, and, years later, he maintains that suicide was never a consideration. "My whole life was about doing everything in my power to *protect* the people I love from harm. Suicide was against everything I stood for, even when I was struggling with the loss of Zeus."

When Tom arrived, he asked Ed to come upstairs. "Eddie, I have somebody coming from a support group to talk to you," he called down to the basement. As Ed made his way, haltingly, up the wooden stairs, two police officers came in through the front door of the split-level ranch and moved up the stairs behind him. When he looked up toward the top of the stairs, there were three more. By the time he finally managed to complete his ascent and step up into the living room, he was completely surrounded by the uniformed police officers. There he was met by a man who introduced himself as a doctor, saying that he was there to do "an evaluation."

Ed knew instantly what was happening. His first thought was that his family had finally gotten tired of him—the inconvenience of him—and that they were going to send him away. He remembers thinking, *My dad wants the house back.*

"I was the one who made the final decision to send Eddie to the hospital," says Bob. "What was I supposed to do? When I'd drop by the house, I'd see Eddie standing in the corner talking to himself. It tore my heart out, but I had to do it." Regardless of the reason, Ed wondered why, as thin and frail as he was, anyone felt the need for such an aggressive display in summoning five police officers. Clearly, they expected a fight.

It's important to remember that Ed's logical mind was always functioning, even as his OCD mind spiraled out of control. His intelligence had not deteriorated, but his body had, and he knew he was in trouble. Physically, there was nothing he could do, but possible escape routes aside, he still felt betrayed that no one had taken the time to simply talk to him about what they felt needed to be done *before* showing up with force, expecting a fight. Why was there no attempt to honor him and treat him as a human being with compassion by talking to him first, the way Ed would have done if roles were reversed?

As Ed looked around at Tommy, Tami, and his father, standing in the living room, he wanted them to explain themselves. Their response is a painful memory that is as fresh today as it was real in that moment. Each of them turned their heads and refused to look him in the eye. Ed resolved in that moment that he would be better than that. He would not give them the fight they were expecting. "I was not going to dishonor my mother, myself, or the memory of Zeus by going out kicking and screaming," says Ed.

After a brief discussion with the doctor, during which Ed was asked by Tommy to "demonstrate" his processes of walking backward and counting, Ed was told by the doctor that an ambulance was already on the way to pick him up. "If the ambulance was already on the way, I knew that a determination of my mental status had been made before the doctor even met me," says Ed. "It had to have been based solely on the word of my brother and, to me, that was just wrong." This served to compound the sense of betrayal Ed felt by his brother, Tom. "I knew I needed help, but they should have talked to me first," says Ed.

Ed asked for a moment to speak to his family alone. There was no arguing or drama during this conversation. Ed told his family he would go and do everything the doctors thought he needed to do to get well, but, in return, he asked that nothing in the basement be touched while he was away—he begged for this reassurance, and according to Tami, he was given the solemn promise by his father that the family would comply with his wishes. At the forefront of Ed's mind was the small plastic bag from the veterinarian that contained clippings of Zeus's hair, and he needed to believe that his only tangible memory of Zeus, along with his countless placeholders of time, would remain untouched until he returned home.

After this reassurance from his father, Ed slowly made his way down the steps to the basement to change into his jeans and put on his shoes. When he was finished, he quietly walked out the side door of the basement and straight into the driveway—as it was the easiest, and most direct route for him to take—and, true to his word, he climbed into the empty vehicle, took a seat in the back, and closed the door.

As Ed sat looking out the small rectangular window of the ambulance door, waiting for the attendants, who were still inside waiting for him to come upstairs, to climb into the cab, there was a sudden commotion outside. He heard one of the officers yell, "He's gone, 'rabbit'!" Apparently, everyone thought he had run away, and they began frantically searching the house's perimeter. But all the while, Ed was sitting in the ambulance doing exactly what he'd promised he would do. The idea that Ed would run away from a promise he'd made was so far out of character for him that he remembers looking around thinking that everyone *else* was crazy. Finally, an officer, who'd been particularly kind to Ed during this process, noticed him peering out the ambulance window and announced, "He's ready to go."

As the ambulance drove away, Ed watched his safe place disappear in the distance, in a scene eerily reminiscent of the day he watched his childhood home disappear from the back window of his father's car after his mother died. From a distance, a heartbroken Tom followed in his car until the ambulance reached the hospital, and he watched in silence as his baby brother climbed out of the ambulance and walked inside.

Ed describes the lobby of the psychiatric ward as a scene from *Terminator 2*—the heavy metal doors with little glass windows up high sliding open and shut, automatically locking behind. He says that almost instantly, he "felt less like a human being." He was asked to remove his shoelaces and belt as he was signed in. Walking down the hall, Ed remembers other mental patients who would come up and try to touch him, and one lady kept screaming, "The Hatfields and McCoys—The Hatfields and McCoys!" Another woman followed him into his room and ran over to his bed to sniff his sheets, frantic as she repeated the words, "chemicals, chemicals!" over and over. In this moment of being forced into the hospital, Ed's obsession shifted from stopping the progression of time, to simply surviving.

There is something uniquely compelling about Ed Zine. It's an odd mixture of overwhelming vulnerability and inner strength, intelligence and grace, determination and will—whatever the formula, it's undeniable even in his weakest state, and during the group counseling sessions he attended throughout the week, he found other patients leaning on him for support.

On one occasion, when he and the other patients were asked to write papers about themselves to read to the group, one young girl who couldn't bring herself to stand up and read, asked Ed to read for her. After he finished, he turned to her at the end, and told her what a good job she did. He says it was the first time in the few days he'd been there that he'd seen her smile.

**THE DAY FOLLOWING HIS ADMISSION,** an intervention meeting was called by the medical team at the hospital, which included Ed, Tom, Tami, their dad, and a couple of Tom and Ed's friends. Ed remembers it as a very contentious meeting. "It was like the Spanish Inquisition. Everyone but Tami was jumping on the verbal bash wagon." Ed remembers his father telling doctors, loud and clear, "If you can't give me my son back healthy, then I don't want him at all. If he's not normal, I don't want him back in my house." Referring back to his notes from that day, psychiatrist Dr. Hoffman says he recorded the fact that Ed's father was "very hostile," and that Ed was gentle, and one of the most reasonable forces in the room.

Dr. Hoffman also goes on to say that while Ed was institutionalized, he wanted to try and get better without the use of medication. He says not only was Ed *not* suicidal, he witnessed almost no sign of Ed's OCD symptoms during this time.

Ed explains it this way: from the moment he agreed to go into the hospital, his OCD shifted from the progression of time, to behaving with dignity and honoring himself. His complete focus was doing everything in his power to make Zeus proud and fulfill the promise he made to his family to do everything he could to try and get better. Ed was bound by this silent code of honor that had been instilled in him as a child, and this is what filled his mind and suppressed the rewinding rituals and compulsions that permeated his brain for so long. This was his method of survival.

During the intervention meeting, Tom placed a stake in the sand and said that if Ed was released before he was better, he would make sure he was put right back in. And, as a cop, Ed knew he had the authority to do it. But Tami sat quietly, helpless to stop the painful exchange among her father and brothers. She also bore her own personal guilt that Ed was here because he had not received the proper care and counseling after their mother's death, and that he had been left alone too long to fend for himself while she was busy trying to care for her own children.

Tami's anguish was compounded by something more—something Ed would soon find out—something she was unable to stop. The moment Ed was taken away to the hospital, their father had broken his promise and cleaned out the basement, dispensing with bags of refuse, including the small plastic bag of Zeus's hair. "It was wrong," she would say years later. "I was there when my father gave his word to Eddie, and he broke it."

According to Tom, everything was black and white in Bob's world, and if you were a real man, you could just stop whatever affliction ailed you by simply making the decision to stop. "My father doesn't understand about mental illness," says Tom. "I remember, one time, hearing him talking about a friend who was an alcoholic and he was, like, 'Why can't they just put down the drink and end it right there?'" But in his defense, Tom says that cleaning the basement of the jars of body waste, the dog hair from Zeus, filthy sheets, magazines, and empty bottles, and shifting things just so he could clean the floors and the furniture and eliminate the stench, was not about spite, but really about ridding his house of the squalor. "My father loves Ed, but he had a lack of compassion for the filth in which he lived," says Tom.

Ed says that after the family meeting, he remembers Dr. Hoffman making the comment to him that he didn't know *how he could* stay sane in that kind of hostile environment. Dr. Hoffman doesn't remember saying those exact words, but he admits it was not an unreasonable thought given that Ed was one of the most rational people in the room that day. By week's end, Ed would check himself out of Pembroke and was given the name by Dr. Hoffman of a clinic where he could receive follow-up care. Otherwise, the stay is noted in the medical records as uneventful.

Ed tried calling home to see if he could find his dad to come pick him up. No one answered, but he was able to pick up messages. One of the messages that came in while he was away was intended for his father from a relative who said, "It's about damn time somebody did it."

He didn't call anyone else in the family to come to pick him up that day. Devastated at the way the whole situation was handled and, under the impression his father had him committed because Ed was an "inconvenience," he called on an old high school friend to come get him.

"Anyone who knows me knows I am not a person who likes to impose on anyone else," says Ed. He'd spent what seemed a lifetime as the youngest kid in the room, trying not to be a bother to anyone who came around because he enjoyed the company of his older siblings and aunts and uncles, and he didn't want to do anything that would make them want to leave sooner than they had to. So the pain of feeling that he, and his disorder, were causing such an imposition on his family caused him terrible grief.

But whatever sadness he was feeling as he left Pembroke Hospital that day was nothing compared to the devastation of walking into his basement to find that his father had broken perhaps the most important promise he had ever made to him. Everything had been moved. The hat on top of his television set, the new bar of Coast soap that sat on top of the fish tank and made the room smell good when it got hot downstairs, dollar bills stacked in the corner, a *Star Wars* magazine he had left on the floor, his dirty T-shirt, Zeus's red mini Kong doggie toy—everything that was so critical to his mental health and the placekeepers of what he considered happier moments—had either been moved or had disappeared all together, having been thrown in the garbage by his father. Most upsetting was the fact that the item at the top of Ed's list, the plastic bag with Zeus's hair, was nowhere to be seen.

Instantly, Ed became nauseous—his world, which had been so carefully created, had physically collapsed—and he felt like he was going to pass out. He was betrayed by the people he loved most. The fingernails against the chalkboard screeched louder than ever. His skin crawled as if a bucket of spiders had been thrown at him and made their way all over his body. Paralysis set in, as his mind fought its way into survival mode—the mode in which he found himself as his space was breeched by all those ill patients the day he *arrived* at Pembroke.

"I have an inner strength that most people do not have, and it's based in honor," says Ed, who clings to the emotion of honor the way a baby clings to his security blanket. It soothes him at times when nothing else in the world can. The idea of doing the right thing, against the odds, embodied by characters through which he lived vicariously in the movies of his childhood, seems to be an almost tangible connection to his mother, bridging that loss and subsequent losses with purpose. It keeps him standing up in the ring, like a prizefighter, as he gets pummeled by one heartbreaking blow after another. It is the emotion that girds him against disappointment and pain.

"Honoring my mother was how I survived her passing, honoring Zeus is how I got through Pembroke, and continuing to honor Zeus's memory was the only way I got through the pain of this experience," says Ed, as he made the decision that however long it took, he would re-create the room as it was—inasmuch as was possible given that so many of his things were discarded. But now, the pushback from Ed's compulsive mind, and the need to rewind, rebounded with a force even greater than before, complicating the process in such a profound way that it would take him months to re-create the room to absolute perfection.

Ed's OCD, where every millimeter matters and every mental and physical rewind must be completed precisely, was enhanced by his photographic memory. Whether he developed this ability over time or it was something he was born with is unknown, but Ed had the rare ability to look around the room that day he arrived back from the hospital, and remember *exactly* where every item had been before he was taken away. But determining where everything had been placed wasn't enough—he had to undergo those same arduous, repetitive, exacting rituals to simply shift things back into their proper place. Just to move Zeus's shampoo bottle that had been sitting on top of the fish tank before he left and moved elsewhere by his dad required countless back and forth maneuvers within fractions of an inch. It took many hours of revision to complete such tasks, and completing these tasks meant when Ed *felt right*. The need to "feel right" is a symptom of OCD that is common in many sufferers, but achieving this feeling isn't an exact science. The sufferer just has to perform tasks and move things about until what Ed describes as the spine-tingling feeling of fingernails against a chalkboard eases.

It would take months to completely fine-tune the basement to a point where Ed's world felt secure again. The replication of the precommitment basement was extraordinary and may sound fascinating—almost triumphant—but the illness was manifesting itself in the most extreme ways.

So, although Ed's family's approach to getting him help may have been the wrong assessment—their efforts were clearly misdirected—there was no question that Ed was ill with OCD; and the rebound effect from the hospitalization, and the betrayal he felt in how his admission was handled, created this desperate and urgent need to "nest," like a woman preparing for the birth of a child. He was preparing his safe haven.

As Ed's illness spiraled to greater depths, Tami, still guilt-stricken, would bear the majority of the responsibility of bringing his food to him, always following his explicit directions for delivery as she came down the steps from the driveway to the basement door. But she would have to hand meals *through* the door. This was his OCD Holy Ground, and no one would be welcomed in it—not until the day that Michael Jenike came along and decided Ed needed a shower—but that day wouldn't come before the person he sought to protect nearly destroyed his will to survive.

*The best thing would be if everything in life was recorded—*
*and God had a big rewind button, so he could say,*
*"Sit in the corner, both of you. Stop being knuckleheads!"*
—ED ZINE

# CHAPTER 9

# History of Pain

◀◀

I HOPE YOU FUCKING DIE!" It was a brutal, heart-stopping ex-
clamation spoken in a moment of blind rage, but Ed's heart
couldn't discern that fact. The careless expletive that tumbled
so easily from his father's lips—words that would eventually be
forgiven, but never forgotten—resulted in an adrenaline-induced
panic, kicking into high gear Ed's time equation obsession and
triggering an explosion of new, more intense rituals.

Bob was upstairs; he had come into the house that morning angry about something, and Ed remembers hearing him open
the door and screaming down the stairs at the top of his lungs.
Within seconds, a black plastic bag, filled with garbage, came
flying down the stairs into the basement. It went boomeranging

off the walls of the landing and straight into the *Running Man* laser disc, which was sitting up against the television set in the exact same place it had been the night that Zeus died. It had taken Ed nearly two months to reset it perfectly in place after his father moved it while he was in the hospital.

The echoes of his father's anger were all too familiar, and the episode, once again, brought Ed right back to the night of his mother's death. Ed was overcome by sudden terror. The irony was that while Ed's obsessive condition would of course bring heartache to *any* parent, Ed's mess, which represented chaos to everyone *but* Ed, ran counter to his ex-wartime marine father's own apparent form of OCD, which, as long as the Zine kids could remember, could only be appeased by a strict regimen of cleanliness and a more traditional definition of order and semblance.

THERE WAS ANOTHER EDWARD ZINE, Ed's grandfather—a bantamweight Lebanese prizefighter from South Boston who became a well-known neighborhood bookie in the forties, when his days in the ring were over. To all who knew him, he bore a strong resemblance to movie star gangster George Raft—always dressed in a sharp suit and vest, starched collars, French-toed shoes, and lots of diamond jewelry. True to form, the elder Edward was not in any way prone to outward displays of affection—quite the opposite, actually. His legacy was his steely toughness, which he passed on to Ed's father, Bob.

But as with many emigrants to America at the time, Edward Zine was forced to make something out of nothing—and *he* did it by being tough. And his parenting was clearly informed by the way in which he beat his own early hardships. Whatever love he felt for his children was shown, not by hugs and kisses, but by the clothes on their backs, the food on their plates, and the strict discipline he instilled in each of his five children. This attitude laid the foundation for the sixteen-year-old Bob who headed off to war—the U.S. Marines took over Edward's child rearing from there.

For men of Bob's generation, the phrase "pull yourself up by the bootstraps" was a way of life. You survived war only by obeying the commands of those surrogate fathers in uniform who commanded you to live a life of unrelenting regimen and strict obedience, and by pushing through whatever pain you experienced with sheer will and determination. Any outward manifestation of feelings and emotions was considered "queer." Military leaders like George Patton, who reportedly slapped two soldiers hospitalized for psychiatric disorders, attached a stigma to mental illness, believing it a sign of weakness and cowardice, and often using it as a threat for possible court-martial. This is the history that Bob carried with him into fatherhood, and the history with which Ed would contend growing up.

Suffice it to say, being raised in a military-style household by an ex-marine who was the son of a prizefighter was far from easy living for a naturally gentle, loving kid. There was little choice but to toughen up and obey the strict rules of his father's command, or suffer the consequences. Ed learned to make his bed with sheets pulled so tight you could bounce a penny off them. He laundered his own clothes, making sure to keep a tight crease in his pants. And most of all, he knew about loyalty. "Semper Fi"—to always be faithful. These were the principles he learned and cherished—and in spite of everything, including Bob's violent episode the night of his wife's death, he maintained his hero status in Ed's eyes. That is, until the Pembroke episode, when his father had him involuntarily committed. The betrayal—the feeling that having control of a clean house was more important than having a healthy son—would leave a lasting impression on Ed and he would, really for the first time, see a tear in his father's moral fabric.

BOB DIDN'T THINK MUCH ABOUT the impact of his actions on his desperately ill son when he stormed furiously out of the house on the day he inadvertently bounced the *Running Man* disc out of place. He wished his son was "normal," but he wasn't, and whatever this OCD was, Bob didn't get it. He had been trained by the military to believe that mental illness was bullshit and that mental weakness just needed a tough guiding hand. It was this unwavering toughness, after all, that brought him home from a war.

Bob didn't understand that *Ed* was now at war—a war between his intellect and his fear of death, taking someone else he loved away from him—and on this particular day, he stormed out without giving Ed closure, the series of repeated words, good-byes, and reassurances that Ed needed at the end of every conversation until he was comfortable that every rewind and replication ritual had been satisfied.

Sick and disoriented from the terror that bound his breath, Ed desperately needed help. Looking at the phone, about fifteen feet down the hall, was like looking at an object through the wrong end of a telescope. For Ed, fifteen feet was the equivalent of fifteen miles for the nonafflicted. Outside, he heard the sounds of the oil delivery truck on the street. He was closer to the basement door than to the phone and, in his panicked state, he thought maybe he could yell for the delivery man to come help. He didn't know exactly what he needed, but Tami, who worked as a teaching assistant at a local school, would know, and she would tell him that everything would be okay. If Ed could just get someone to call her, she would come and tell him that everything would be okay. With nothing on but sweatpants, Ed made his way outside the basement door and up the cold, wet steps in his stocking feet to search for help. He focused on memorizing the movements so he could retrace them, backward, when he came back inside:

*First step with right foot . . . left foot . . . make sure legs are perfectly perpendicular, step back and step forward . . . don't think about cold . . . repeat steps until reaching top, pay attention to step around brick . . . don't think about cold, move right foot around bend, make sure not to step on little thing about six inches high . . . swing left foot around, keep body at a slight angle, not too much . . . right foot . . . left foot . . . right foot . . . stop at paint spots on asphalt where somebody sprayed paint . . . breathe . . . check hands, fingers locked . . . yell for help . . . no response . . . keep moving . . . move right foot, left foot. Don't think about cold. Yell for help, again. Freeze. Lock legs. Rewind. Commit the whole process to memory. Yell for help again.*

Ed's voice was as frail and thin as the rest of his shivering body, and it took a while before the Wynne Oil delivery man was able to hear the high-pitched, dog-whistle cries of "Help . . . hello . . . help!" As the truck driver pulled up in front of Ed's house and saw the sight of the sickly, bare-chested young man standing in his stocking feet in the puddles of rain from the night before, he jumped out of his cab and ran over to see what he could do to help. Ed struggled to recount the story of his illness and the fight with his father, and he asked the stranger to get a message to his sister at school to come help.

The gentleman from Wynne Oil climbed back into his truck, got on the CB, called his home base, and they, in turn, were able to get a message to Tami at school. The delivery man came back and waited with Ed and tried to talk him into going back inside to get warm, but it was useless. The only thing Ed could do was rock back and forth from his heels to the balls of his feet, shivering from the cold, and count to himself while he rewound the morning's events in his head. As impossible as it seems, the obsession that racked his mind with worry was the fear that his father would die because the closing rituals of their good-bye had not been completed. In a relationship that was incredibly harsh, and often cruel, the love between them never subsided, and regardless of how Bob viewed Ed's illness, it was fueled by the need to keep his father alive and well.

Ed's greatest need at the height of any OCD crisis, as is the case with the majority of sufferers, is reassurance. It is a short-term solution that actually reinforces OCD, because the more reassurance one gets, the more one needs. But even for family members—*especially* for family members—who are educated about the cycle and the long-term benefits of *not* indulging this extreme need for constant reassurance, it is of course difficult to ignore the short-term benefits of giving the person they love relief from the obvious pain.

When Tami got the call that her brother was in trouble, she recalls her first reaction as, "Oh, my God, what has Dad done to provoke this?" After a quick call to Deena asking her to pick up the kids after school, she rushed over to the house where Ed was petrified—almost literally. It was a heartbreaking sight as she pulled into the driveway, "Ed standing there shirtless in the middle of winter, rocking back and forth. I knew right then that he was stuck."

"Stuck" meant hours of reassurances and calming words that would bring Ed back from the edge of whatever terrifying preci-pice he was overlooking at that moment. Although Ed's require-ments for appeasement were very specific, compliance with his requests necessitated love and support to work through the anxi-ety. In this case, he needed patience from someone he believed in so that he could begin taking steps back toward the house. Ed had been standing in one place so long that his legs started to give out underneath him and, automatically, Tami reached out to grab his arm and try to steady him, but it only made things worse, sending Ed into a spiral of thousands upon thousands of rewind-ing rituals within rituals to erase the human contact that had, by this point, become so incredibly uncomfortable for him.

It took nearly six hours of placid words for Tami to get Ed to begin making the physical move backward into the basement. By this time, he was frozen stiff—still bare chested, with soak-ing wet feet—making his movements even harder to control, and thus more difficult to replicate perfectly.

"While Tami was talking to me, I finally started moving," re-members Ed, "swaying back and forth and back and forth for the counting that I was doing in my head. As vehicles passed by, I'd have to wait for another one to go past for an even number, just so I could start to go in reverse, and walk backwards, which means I was standing in one spot, and had to move both legs left to right, perpendicular to each other, and then step backward and forward. That's just one movement. I had to step back in the same spot, exactly, and step forward again. That is a ritual, and I had to reverse it. It was like having a videotape that you watch in reverse. If I stepped back, I had to watch and see if I deviated from the course just a little bit, because if I did, it wasn't correct; it's not the same forward motion that you went, and the same parallel lines that you went back. There was so much pressure to get that line exact, without leaning. It's all about timing while you try to lock the left leg so the right can go back in the same spot. You go forward and touch and you go backward and touch, making sure that you don't hear noises that can freeze you, and lock you. Sometimes, when a car went by, my leg would freeze, and I would have to hold it in midair, and it could be another twenty minutes to an hour before another car went by and I could move again."

When Ed finally got back to the bottom of the basement steps and walked backward across the threshold, Tami was not allowed to follow him inside. Even after all of those hours in and out of the cold, she had to walk around to the front of the house and wait until Ed crossed back through the basement to stand at the door that separated the upstairs from the basement so she could listen to the strict routine that his OCD required for her to unlock the front door. It went like this:

*Put the key in the lock, turn to the right, then turn to the left.*
*Repeat this process four times. Walk through the door, open*
*and close the door behind two, four, or eight times, according*
*to whatever "felt right" to Ed as he listened from downstairs.*
*Get the key from the living room that will open the dead bolt*
*to the basement door. Remember not to say the word dead; use*

*the word freath. Insert key into the "freath bolt" turn to the*
*right, and then to the left. Repeat four times. Open the door,*
*close the door, repeat two, four, or eight times as determined*
*by Ed who is standing on the other side of the door—if he is*
*not in "perfect position" on the other side of the door, the entire*
*process will have to begin again.*

It takes unconditional love to accept someone with OCD, and Tami knows this. Ed's father's history precluded him, like so many families of OCD sufferers, from *trying* to understand the mental illness that turned his son into someone he could no longer recognize. Bob *would* eventually alter his perspective to successfully confront Ed's illness, but not before things got much worse.

# CHAPTER 10

# A Different Kind of Doctor

A CCORDING TO ARNOLD HIATT, FORMER chairman of the Stride Rite Corporation and current chairman of the Stride Rite Foundation, "Michael [Jenike] is one of the more remarkable pioneers in medicine, but he doesn't share the same self-importance of many of his peers."

Despite his groundbreaking approach to OCD and his sick patients, Michael simply describes himself as an imperfect man with sensible ideals about what is central to his responsibilities as a physician. But, despite his tendency to break with protocol and manifest his frustration with politics and the current health-care system, he is an optimist. He believes if he does the right thing for his patients, everything will work out for the best. This is the thinking that allows him to buck the profit-driven systems of health-care management because not only is he, quite literally, among the best in the world, the time and effort he has put in to his research and treatment in the area of obsessive-compulsive disorder has returned to him tenfold in the form of financial support from those he's helped. With the papers he's published and the public accolades he's received, Michael's profile has grown and his practice has attracted the attention of certain high-profile patients. These patients have in turn helped fund projects like the OCD Institute, which provides residential treatment for desperately ill patients who, even with the support of their families, cannot properly function on the outside and benefit from the intensive round-the-clock treatment they receive from a staff of trained psychiatrists, psychologists, and behavioral therapy counselors. The support has also enabled Michael to bill the clients who can afford his services and waive the bill for those who can't. He is a compassionate clinician who ignores the bureaucratic health-care system, which dictates that he can only spend fifteen-minute intervals with his patients, steadfastly refusing to make a rapid diagnosis or prescribe medicine or therapy until he is absolutely certain he fully comprehends a particular patient's needs.

Before coming to work at the OCD Institute, Diane Davey, Program Manager and Administrative Director, heard comments around the hospital suggesting that Michael was "a hothead, someone who flipped out for no reason at all." In fact, when she was considering the job, she was warned by acquaintances at work about his reputation. But being offered the chance to work in the start-up phase of the Institute and tackle the challenges that awaited presented an exciting opportunity. So, for the first year they worked together, she took the precaution of handling Michael gently, just in case the rumors turned out to be credible.

In time, however, Diane came to know Michael quite differently. "Michael marches to the beat of his own drum, and he's not intimidated by anyone. But I didn't find him to be contrary at all," she remembers. "If he is angry about something, he always has a good reason."

Michael reserves his temper and indignant behavior for insurance companies as he fights to convince them of the importance of specific treatments and hospital stays they won't cover. He is bewildered by what he calls "a system of unqualified strangers making critical decisions about patients on whom they've never laid eyes, and determining which physician treatment plans are 'not medically necessary.'" He believes it is *his* responsibility to evaluate his patients, "find out who they are, where they are, and what's going on, *then* ask what they want out of life and how I can help them get to where they want to go."

On one occasion, Diane had spent time coaching Michael for the insurance review that he was about to undertake regarding a patient who required a series of cognitive and behavioral therapies, making diplomatic suggestions about how he might approach some of the questions he was going to be asked. However, during the *actual* meeting, Diane heard something slam against the wall between their offices. Apparently, to counter Michael's argument for residential care so that the therapies could be most effectively performed, the insurance reviewer decided to give Michael an education on the various drugs that were now available on the market for the treatment of OCD, unaware that Michael had *conducted* the drug companies' studies for the very same medications. It was at this point that Michael's temper got the best of him, and he pulled the phone off the desk and threw it across the room. End of meeting.

Michael does understand *why* insurance companies have cracked down on psychiatrists over the past fifteen years. Abuse of the system used to be rampant. In fact, in the early days of his residency, Michael watched many analytical psychiatrists take advantage of the reimbursement system when all they had to do to get paid was submit a bill. Psychiatric *residents* were, at the time, encouraged to enter psychotherapy for long periods of time for *educational* purposes. Their supervisors wanted them to "learn about therapy" via the process of being evaluated themselves. The psychiatrists would then bill residents' insurance companies to the tune of thousands and thousands of dollars for each resident, wasting money that should have gone to *real* patient care.

For years after he completed his residency, Michael believed that the goal of many hospitals still was to keep patients as long as possible in order to make the most money. But as insurance companies tried to get a handle on costs, they implemented a policy whereby a lump sum was to be paid in its entirety upon admission that *they* deemed was appropriate for a patient's care, regardless of the length of stay. And of course, today, the money doled out by insurance companies often isn't even close enough to cover the stay a patient might require to make a full recovery. For Michael, it has been maddening.

But at the OCD Institute, where Michael is director, he's implemented what he believes is the most sensible system for his patients. "We do what is clinically indicated," says Michael, who emphasizes that a person's insurance doesn't dictate his length of stay. His entire staff enforces this patient-friendly policy.

In its first year of operation, based on this pragmatic model—during a time when money was drying up for long-term psychiatric care hospitals—the OCD Institute broke even, which actually made it successful. And since it opened, the Institute has more than made its bottom line, actually doing as well as most other groups within the hospital. Arnold Hiatt, who provided funding for the original launch, says it was clear that Massachusetts General Hospital was not prepared, initially, to invest any funds in a project it considered to be experimental, which this was, so he agreed to underwrite any deficits for a period of years. "I got off easy," he says.

For the most part, Michael admittedly does not bother to bill the patients he sees in his clinic at Massachusetts General Hospital because the paperwork he needs to provide the insurance company is just too cumbersome. Michael estimates that about 20 percent of physicians' time is being taken away from their patient care because they are trying to meet insurance companies' and hospitals' administrative paperwork demands. As for those patients Michael bills privately, he always adds a note, "If this bill is too much, just pay what you want."

Part of the solution, he suggests, would be to create a standardized form to file patient insurance claims, saving doctors countless hours of work. Not only that, he says, if the hospital administrative processes within every hospital were standardized across the country, there would be massive savings within the health-care system that would put money back into covering the costs of actual patient care.

**IN THE EARLY DAYS OF** his career, Michael routinely gave speeches on behalf of drug companies, talking about all the medicines that were useful in the treatment of OCD. He felt these events provided a valuable platform for providing physicians and other treatment providers with an education on the disorder. But he then began getting pressured to use their slides and promote individual drugs. So in 1990, he wrote an op-ed piece in the *New England Journal of Medicine* opposing the relationships between physicians and pharmaceutical companies and, in practicing what he preached, immediately stopped taking drug company money for talks, slicing his income by at least $50,000 a year.

Patricia Perkins, former executive director of the Obsessive Compulsive Foundation, says, "Michael doesn't pontificate, he simply leads by example." More than anything, Michael wants young doctors to know that they have an obligation to spend as much time with a patient as is required to make him or her better—be it fifteen minutes or an hour, insurance company mandates be damned. He feels that insurance companies are, directly or indirectly, affecting the training of future physicians who are becoming all too familiar with the time crunch. He maintains that "the more resourceful among the young physicians will figure out a way to be flexible, and take care of their patients effectively." But he worries about those who will religiously follow the authority figure in charge and the rules that do not make the best sense for their patients.

Michael believes it is important for doctors to give away their time and expertise to people who need it. He makes himself accessible to patients all over the country by publicizing his private e-mail address and answering an average of three hundred e-mails a day. He actively seeks out support groups and OCD chat rooms, often dropping in spontaneously to listen to what patients have to say, participate in the discussion, and answer questions they might have. And he doesn't make any attempts to hide his twisted and irreverent humor in dealing with OCD patients and often uses it to lighten the mood and break the awful anxiety that comes along with the disorder. Wendy Mueller, who heads up an online group, says that Michael has been visiting for several years and keeps a file of Michael's most memorable responses—many of which demonstrate his wantonly humorous approach:

*One woman writes: "I have this new worry about getting stuck with an AIDS needle at the movie theater. I have a red scab on the back of my leg thinking that's where the needle got me . . . I wish I never went to the theater. It's my fault."*

*Michael's response: "Ahhhh . . . so many of you fear getting AIDS from a needle in a movie seat! I should develop butt armor. If we could get the 'fatal needle-in-the-butt' obsession going among the six million members of the OCD community, I could make a fortune. I could call my new butt armor psycho-anal-lysis."*

# CHAPTER 11

# Ed's Faith Regained

⏪

E**D'S HAD AN AVERSION TO** doctors since the first time his dad hauled him into therapy after his mother died. He never forgot the attitude of the therapist who looked down at the plumber and his kids, as if he were somehow better. So as Ed sat across the room from Michael during their first meeting in the spring of 1996, he was watching for any signs of that same "doctor's ego." "I'd had too many experiences where it was, 'me doctor, you patient—me talk, you listen,'" says Ed. Ed felt it was important that a doctor take the time to get to know individuals from when they were young, not just from when they were sick. He goes on to say, "Dr. Jenike wasn't like that. He didn't talk down to me, he talked to me like I was a human being."

Ed reiterated the integral importance of Michael's trustworthiness, and he was assured that anything he said would be kept confidential, even from his family. But as he watched Michael walk down the steps to the front door of the split-level ranch, and outside to face his family, who were anxiously waiting for an assessment, the five-month-old fears caused by the Pembroke conspiracy rushed back to him.

**TOM HAD DISCOVERED MICHAEL PURELY** by accident as he was channel surfing. A frequent guest expert on news shows and the daytime circuit, Michael was talking about OCD. After speaking with Tami, the two made plans to reach out to Dr. Jenike right away.

These were the days before widespread Internet access, and it wasn't easy to track someone down, but Tami's homework finally led her to Massachusetts General Hospital, where the switchboard operator then transferred her to Michael's secretary, Mary. Mary responded to Tami's initial inquiry with the standard protocol and sent her a big manila envelope stuffed with pamphlets about OCD and the OCD Institute. The full extent of Ed's disorder was not disclosed at that time.

When the packet finally arrived, it was like a lightbulb went off—it was as if everything was written specifically about Ed. Knowledge is power, and the family had never been given this much information about OCD before. Ed wasn't an anomaly, there were others like him, and Dr. Jenike and his treatment facility offered hope for Ed. But their chances of getting him to Boston were slim to none.

Tami persisted in a way that was out of character for her—she refused to let this opportunity to get Ed help pass by. She picked up the phone, got Mary on the line again, and told her the whole story.

Mary was one of the few people who knew about Michael's struggle with posttraumatic stress disorder. She was instrumental in quietly helping him navigate his workload efficiently during that time, and she continued to feel protective of him as his schedule rebounded back to normal. But a "normal" schedule for Michael really meant "overload," and as much as she knew he needed all of his free time for himself, she also knew the minute he heard Ed's story, he would be off to the Cape.

True to form, the moment Michael received the note from Mary, he sent a message back to the family promising that he would come as soon as he could arrange his schedule.

**AS ED WATCHED MICHAEL THROUGH** the large picture window in the living room, he prepared himself for a letdown, anxiously waiting to see if Michael would cave to the pressure from his family and betray his trust, as his family had when he was shipped off to Pembroke. But Michael stopped for only a brief second, acknowledged them with what appeared to be a "goodnight," and was on his way. Even though it was perfectly natural for Tom, Tami, and Ed's father to try and bombard Michael with questions about what had transpired, he kept his promise, and answered simply, "I will not betray Ed's confidence."

Ed couldn't hear the words Michael spoke to his family, but he instinctively knew from the short exchange that he'd kept his word and thus was a man of honor. In that simple moment, Michael had gained enough of Ed's trust that he would be allowed, albeit cautiously, into the circle of his torturous life.

Just that spring, Michael opened the doors of the OCD Institute—which, as it happened, was the first residential facility in the United States designed exclusively for the treatment of obsessive-compulsive disorder—as part of McLean Hospital and Massachusetts General Hospital. He'd pushed the idea for several years, but it was repeatedly shut down by the hospital's administration after being labeled unprofitable. The OCD Institute only became a reality when Arnold Hiatt, CEO of the Stride Rite Foundation, supported the vision and funded the project's start-up.

During this period, psychiatrists and psychologists all over the country were actively engaged in what some call a professional turf war over the issue of whether medicine or behavioral therapy was the best treatment for OCD. Michael stayed out of the fray, steadfastly pursuing what he believed was the more successful middle ground—a combination of both medicine and behavioral therapy. He used this approach in intensive, around-the-clock treatment at the OCD Institute for those patients severely affected by the disorder, and the results were good. Ultimately, Jenike was credited as one of the top leaders in the universally accepted approach to treatment for OCD.

After only one meeting, Michael immediately felt Ed could seriously benefit from the kind of intensive care he would receive at the OCD Institute. But it was painfully clear to him that there was no way Ed was going to willingly leave the basement of his home, especially with the trauma he suffered from his recent hospitalization. "Psychiatric hospitalization is a huge blow to one's self-esteem," says Michael. "Most severely ill OCD patients hospitalized in general psychiatric units are not helped if the unit does not treat the patient specifically for OCD, or it is not behaviorally oriented. Some patients even get worse." But Michael also knew that Ed wasn't ready to give up control of the environment that had been violated while he was in the hospital. Going to the OCD Institute was simply out of the question.

**SOMETHING ABOUT THIS KID STRUCK** a deep nerve in Michael. As Ed talked about his preoccupation with death, and all the rituals he performed to stop the progression of time, there was a subtext of honor and trust woven into every story, and as desperately ill as he was, he somehow held on to the slim hope that everything would turn out okay. Maybe, subconsciously, Michael was reminded of all the young men Ed's age who served in Vietnam—so many who brought that same sliver of optimism and naive militaristic code of honor to battle—so many who lost the fight.

Ed's war raged inside his mind. Unlike a lot of the young people Michael encountered during family-initiated interventions, he wasn't hostile. But he was unequivocal in what he was willing to do—he would talk to Michael, but he would not leave the house, he would not take prescription medication, and he would not trust anyone to tell him what to do.

With these restrictions, there was little Michael could do to mount an effective plan for treatment. The most he could hope for as he left that day was to keep open the lines of communication, and in time find an opportunity to reintroduce the traditional two-pronged treatment option of medicine and behavioral therapy.

Over the next two months, as Ed struggled with the demands of his OCD, he began to reach out to Michael over the phone. The time equation that formed the initial basis of his disorder was splintering off into a variety of manifestations with increasing frequency. From counting and checking, to contamination and hoarding, the more Ed tried to keep up with his obsessive and compulsive behaviors, the worse they got. He would find himself unable to move from the bathroom for three hours, or he got stuck on a particular number, counting in even numbers and having to repeat the process over hundreds and thousands of times. Thoughts of his mother were recurring with greater frequency, and he couldn't get certain scenes out of his head. His bedsores needed tending, and he didn't understand why he got them or how to make them go away. "I needed to have constant contact," says Ed, "and Dr. Jenike gave his home and cell numbers to Tami and Tom. They would come over and dial the number for me to save me the hours it would take for me to do it." When they came, Ed wouldn't have to walk so far because they would bring the phone to him, which would eliminate his need to repeat dial and stand frozen in one place while he waited for the callbacks.

Typically, Ed would have to make at least four callbacks for every phone call he made, but Michael refused to accommodate that need and allowed him only the one additional callback necessary to make it an even number. "He wasn't trying to control or manipulate me," says Michael, who admits that most therapists typically wouldn't give any concession at all. "Ed *needed* to make it an even number, and I was willing to be flexible to that point."

As the frequency of their conversations increased, Michael sprinkled in information about OCD, and the various treatment modalities. "He broke it down for me, gradually, educating me about OCD without making demands of me and increasing my anxiety," says Ed. "He continually reminded me that OCD is a disorder, it's not who I am as a person. He took a very holistic approach to my care, and when things got too intense, he would lighten the mood with his humor."

For example, if they were talking about bedsores and the importance of good hygiene, and Ed started to get anxious, Michael would say something like, "Listen, stinky, you and I both know you're going to have to take a shower *sometime*." Or, if Ed would try to keep Michael on the phone too long, he would cut him off by saying, "Look, gruesome, it's time to get your smelly ass off the phone, I'm busy." Ed says if anyone else had dared to comment about his physical appearance, he wouldn't appreciate it, "but he approached it in a way that allowed me to acknowledge the situation without making me feel bad about myself."

Michael's transparency set him apart from everyone else in Ed's world. There were no history, no bias, no behind-the-scenes "conspiracy" plots. Michael was up front and had no agenda other than for Ed to get well. He chose not to charge Ed for his time, so money wasn't the ulterior motive. He wasn't being controlled or influenced by members of Ed's family to do what *they* thought was right. Michael's interaction with Ed was based on pure, unadulterated compassion. And as harsh as that may sound, given the fact that Tom, Tami, and Deena cared about Ed, and did what they could to help meet the demands of his OCD, the bottom line was that Ed felt he couldn't trust anyone to operate in his absolute best interest—there were always other influences in their decision making—whether it was the house, his father, or the fact that his OCD was too invasive in their lives and they wanted a quick fix. Michael became the only person Ed could fully believe in—but he'd been burned enough to know that he could never trust *anyone* completely—except himself.

As their working relationship developed, and Michael sensed Ed's comfort level increase, he eased back into the subject of drug therapy. According to Ed, Michael was very methodical in laying out all the pros and cons of any medicine that he thought would be beneficial, and then he turned the decision over to Ed. "It was always, 'I think this could help you, here's why, and what do *you* think?'" says Ed. "Never, 'you *need* to do this.'"

Most of the drugs involved in the treatment of OCD are antidepressants. The six drugs shown to be effective in double-blind studies are Luvox, Prozac, Zoloft, Celexa, Paxil, and Anafranil, but, according to Michael, it remains unclear as to why these particular drugs help OCD. Each has potent effects on a particular neurotransmitter, or chemical messenger, in the brain called serotonin. Serotonin is one of several neurotransmitter chemicals that nerve cells in the brain use to communicate with one another. Its uptake and release affects much of our mental life, including OCD and depression. The time it takes for these medications to take effect averages ten to twelve weeks, with the dose often having to be adjusted upward to get the best results.

By summer's end, Ed made the decision to give drug therapy a try. "It was a very big deal for me," says Ed. "I really wanted to get better, but it was also important to me that Dr. Jenike *knew* I was trying."

By the fall of 1996, Michael's twofold treatment plan was in motion when he added cognitive behavioral therapy (CBT) to the mix. With Ed's permission, Michael invited a highly respected behavioral therapist with whom he worked to join him in a house call to the Cape to begin CBT.

CBT involves two main components: exposure, and response (ritual) prevention. The idea is to have the patient repeatedly confront a fearful situation *without* giving in to the ritualistic response that is provoked by the anxiety it causes. The repetition of exposures is done until the fear diminishes, the anxiety abates, and the rituals correspondingly decrease or are entirely vanquished. The successful outcome of this therapy is called habituation.

During exposure therapy, the therapist's job is to push the patient's anxiety limits, and there are no reassurances given that everything will be okay, because it would be detrimental to the process. CBT can be an excruciatingly painful, and often contentious, experience as the patient is caught between the demands of his or her OCD and the therapist.

The initial goal was to try and get Ed to walk upstairs and go outside while minimizing the number of counting rituals he performed as he was doing it. But Ed continued to try to move forward up the stairs until he performed every count, until every accidental touch was accompanied by the even number of re-touches, until every movement of his feet to the right, then left, was replayed to his OCD satisfaction. "I kept trying to tell him that I couldn't do what he was asking me to do, and I felt so much pressure," recalls Ed. "I was consumed with meeting the demands of my OCD, and the instructions sounded, to me, like gibberish.

"I wanted them to know that I didn't have control, and that behavioral therapy made me feel uncomfortable." Although Ed understands the concept of behavioral therapy, he says, "Who's to say that the doctor knows when you're ready to face those fears—only in progressing discussions can the doctor and patient figure these things out."

According to Michael, "It works for a lot of patients, but it was clear that we were not going to be able to give Ed a bunch of rules and tell him what he had to do."

Ed recalls, "I knew what I could do and what I couldn't do, and I didn't want to be made to feel bad for not being able to control my OCD in that particular moment."

It was a setback for sure, but Michael was not going to give up on the idea of behavioral therapy just because this first attempt didn't turn out well. "I got all wrapped up in trying to figure out how to get him out of that hell," says Michael, who was also dealing with changes in Ed's prescription regimen. Ed was struggling with reactions to the medicine—his selective serotonin reuptake inhibitors (SSRIs)—that included migraines, muscle spasms, nightmares, and nausea. "The problem," says Ed, "wasn't a lack of serotonin that caused my OCD. Mine was memory based, and they don't make a pill to erase memory. So I needed the two C's—closure to the problem, and coping skills so I wouldn't regress."

As obvious as it seems, in retrospect, that the loss of Ed's mother was at the root of his OCD, it was only over a long period of time that he would reveal his most painful childhood experiences to Michael. "The more I was with him," says Ed, "the more easily I could explain what I was feeling, and he would give me the medical explanation, so I could begin to understand the connection." But it wasn't just the loss of his mother; it was everything that loss represented in terms of uncertainty, and the constant shifting from one place to another. OCD thrives on the stress of transition and uncertainty. Ed's need to repeat and rewind was his way to create a sense of security and certainty that he felt he could control.

# CHAPTER 12

# A Step Forward

B Y MAY OF 1997, MICHAEL was starting to run out of medicines that he could try with Ed, and he decided to reintroduce the idea of CBT. His oldest daughter, Lisa, was a behavioral
therapy counselor at the OCD Institute and, like Michael, has a
very gentle and warm demeanor. He brought her to the Cape on
Memorial Day with the express purpose of introducing her to Ed.
If the meeting went well, he would pay Lisa privately to have her
make the three-hour trip to Cape Cod once a week to work with
him on her day off. Joining them were two former patients from
the OCD Institute who had successfully completed CBT and
were now doing well. Michael planned to cheerlead Ed through
to the next phase of his treatment.

Ed stood anxiously behind the basement door and refused to come upstairs. He was ashamed of the way he looked and didn't want to meet anyone. It was a tense moment, as Ed felt the pressure of wanting to please Michael, not wanting him to leave, and feeling humiliated by his OCD. Michael broke the tension by telling Ed to "get his gruesome ass in the shower and wash off the stank." Completely disarmed by Michael's humor, Ed suddenly agreed to do it, on the condition that Michael would talk him through it. Not only was this a huge turning point because he hadn't showered in almost two years, but he was also going to allow Michael to come into the basement for the first time. Ed was caught up in the moment, ready to show Michael how much he appreciated everything he'd done for him. But first, he told everyone to wait upstairs while he got ready.

Michael waited upstairs for nearly two hours while Ed walked backward to the bathroom, pulled out his hair clippers, and began to buzz off all of his long, dirty, matted hair. *This is good*, he thought, as he methodically created a mental image of each section of hair he shaved. Unable to physically rewind the event, he was compiling a videotape of the process that he would rewind mentally when everyone was gone, and he was alone. Reimagining an event was what he calls "a cheap substitute" for manifestly reversing an action, but it was the least he could do to keep his obsessions at bay and hold time in its place. As he watched himself in the mirror, and he struggled to lift each lock of hair and touch it with the edge of the clippers, Ed recalls, "The hounds of OCD were trying to get loose in my head." Pushing back the tormenting forces of his illness, he focused on what he looked like when his body was in perfect shape at Clemson, and on that clean, all-American image that he wanted to show Michael and

Lisa. And when he was done, he moved backward to the bottom of the steps and called Michael into the basement.

**WITH HIS HEAD SHORN, ED** issued instructions for Michael to come downstairs. Step *here, don't touch that, move this way, watch your hands, be careful!* Ed was not only anxious about what Michael might accidentally touch, or move, he was also extremely embarrassed by his controlled environment and wondered if it would be too much for Michael.

Michael moved slowly, focused on the fact that he was entering Ed's sacred world, but as he descended into the basement, he had to force himself to breathe through his mouth so that he wouldn't throw up. The stench was unbearable. Michael had been exposed to these smells before from the distance of the living room, but in close quarters, it was excruciating.

As Michael examined the dark, stifling chaos of Ed's OCD world for the first time, his calm face belied the horror of what he was seeing. There were sticky brown rings all over the linoleum floor where Gatorade bottles filled with urine had overflowed and left their marks, while dozens more bottles half filled with yellow waste sat open. The rich smell of days-old urine played havoc in the atmosphere as it blended with the rotting feces in Ziploc bags stacked in green trash bags. The sheets on Ed's bed were green and slimy from body waste, and crumbs of food waste lay on the floor near the end of the bed, while everything in the room was covered with dust. Lying on the floor were food wrappers and stacks of *Star Wars* magazines. And in the middle of this war zone were dozens of sketchbooks lying around with brilliantly drawn pictures.

In an effort to dispel the tension, Michael said, as nonchalantly as possible, "Look at you, my boy, you look like a human being!"

Ed smiled, proudly, and continued walking backward in the direction of the bathroom. Michael asked about the drawings, as Ed made mental notes of Michael's every move toward him so he could mentally rewind the entire event later that night when he was alone. Between his own carefully placed footsteps, and the mental rewinding of every sentence, it wasn't easy to hold a conversation with Michael, but he was trying. The drawings, he explained, haltingly, were his. His art was the one thing in his life that OCD did not control. For reasons he could not explain, he could express himself in his drawings without having to count, or retrace the moves of his pencil. *Wait, was the big toe of my left foot pointed to the right, or to the left?* he wondered suddenly. Distracted, he had to start all over again. *Left foot up, left foot down, toe in, toe out, toe in, toe out.* Getting back to the bathroom that day, and having Michael downstairs in his environment, created almost as much anxiety as the actual idea of taking the shower itself.

Encouraged by Michael's response to his shaved head, Ed moved back into position in front of the mirror before heading into the shower and prepared to dry-shave his long, straggly beard. The simple act of retrieving his razor took more than twenty minutes, as he carefully maneuvered his fingers to ensure the minimum number of touches of the sink, and the razor itself, because each touch required countless retouches until everything felt right so he could proceed.

Layers of hair came off with each rough stroke of the blade, along with layers of dead skin, and Ed's anxiety increased with each stroke of the blade. Ed could hear Michael talking to him, but the words came in and out of focus, echoing in his brain like the sounds of a bad dream—the voice of his OCD was trying to drown him out. He worked hard to stay focused on moving across his face, memorizing each move, and each fallen chunk of hair that fell into the sink.

*Count—remember—count—don't end on an odd number— how many times did the blade move down my skin, how many times did I hit the razor against the side of the sink, how many times . . . how many times? Even numbers—keep counting— remember the order in which everything happened . . . how will the water feel against my skin? Is Michael okay? Where is the soap? What is Lisa doing upstairs? Is she touching anything? Are there spiders in the shower? Checklist where family members are this weekend—are they all wearing their seat belts? Are they all okay? . . . Will the Running Man laser disc at the bottom of the stairs get bumped when Michael goes back up into the living room? Are my fingers touching anything but the handle of the razor? How will I undress?*

In almost a stream of consciousness, Ed forced himself to talk to Michael, giving a running commentary of what he was doing, what he was thinking, and why. He peppered the commentary with requests to Michael to remember not to touch the walls or bump into anything. "I was fighting with my OCD because my OCD is controlling. I'm fighting my own mind making sure to not let my OCD control other people. So I was going through all of these separate hells just to deal with shaving and taking a shower."

When he finished shaving, before taking off his clothes, Ed asked Michael if he would get into the shower and check it for spiders and cobwebs. He needed to know that there was nothing in there that would touch his skin. As Michael stood inside the shower, fully clothed, Ed made another request. Would he also please remove the bar of soap from the inset dish in the wall and hand it to him when he was ready? This would prevent Ed from having to risk touching the dish and having to worry about accompanying contamination and touching rituals. Michael agreed, and when he was finished, he stepped out into the hallway to give Ed privacy to undress.

The bottoms of the white tube socks Ed wore were grimy and filthy. Taking them off was a ritual within a ritual where he had to not bump his hands into any other part of his body. The removal of Ed's light gray Tiger Paw sweatpants and the dirty white Clemson T-shirt yellowed from months of perspiration was equally daunting. Each piece of clothing represented experiences that had been lived while wearing them—movies watched— time kept in place—safety. Taking them off irrevocably changed those experiences in Ed's mind. Removal represented a shift—a move forward—and he would have to take them off carefully, and remember exactly each move he made so he could later erase the entire event in his OCD mind, as if it had never happened.

From the hallway, Michael continually assessed his patient's mental and emotional status, as he tried to keep the mood light, prodding Ed with humor. "Listen, gruesome," he teased, adopting various similar nicknames for Ed over time, "I sure hope people don't get the wrong idea when they find out we've taken a shower together."

Finally undressed, Ed carefully moved the shower curtain

back with the tips of two fingers so no other parts of his body were touched, then moved to the back of the shower stall. He closed the curtain and asked Michael to come in and reach through the front of the curtain and turn on the water. This small act that would take Michael seconds would shave off as much as thirty minutes to an hour of touching and retouching rituals for Ed had he done it himself.

Michael complied, carefully checking the water temperature to make sure that it wasn't too hot, or too cold, so that it wouldn't shock Ed's body. He stepped back and encouraged Ed to step into the water when he was ready.

Ed moved tentatively toward the faucet and slowly reached his hand into the water. Every pulse of the tepid liquid felt like shards of glass against his skin. The pain was physical and mental, as he struggled to reconcile the uncontrollable feeling of time moving forward in a way that he could not easily recapture. How could he possibly count every drop of water hitting his flesh? He couldn't. It was impossible. His mind raced to find a solution. He'd come this far, and he didn't want to disappoint himself, or Michael, by quitting. Count . . . recapture . . . count. If he could count the number of seconds the water hit each part of his body—hand . . . water . . . one, two, three, four . . . then imagine the water returning from his skin to the faucet and flowing back down into the pipes—that would work. He could live with that erasure of time. Okay, breathe. Now, he could proceed, and move his arm into the water, then his leg, then his entire body. His photographic memory would allow him the comfort of being able to recall each movement with precision.

"Are you okay?" Michael asked from the other side of the room.

"Yes," answered Ed—he was okay now.

"Now, scrub that ass!" Michael said jokingly to lighten the moment as he thrust his hand through the curtain and handed Ed the bar of soap he'd been holding.

Ed recalls laughing so hard that he almost slipped backward and fell. "All I could think of to say back was that Telly Savalas line from *Kojak*— 'Who loves ya, baby!'"

But the laughter soon subsided as Ed's OCD reprimanded him for taking leave of his neuroses. *Stay focused*, it reminded him, *don't lose count, don't touch the wall, the handles of the faucet with your back or legs, don't forget your movements, or time will slip forward without your memory, and loved ones will die*. The ominous mood shift was made more manageable because Michael was on the other side of the room, offering constant moral support, and an unending stream of jokes.

Michael's encouragement enabled Ed to finish his shower in less than two hours—a minor miracle given the fact that he had been known to get stuck in one place, unable to move, for several hours at a time—but there was still much work to be done. Now that he was clean, he had to get out of the shower without contaminating himself by accidentally touching the shower curtain or the walls. He had to dry himself off, and the towel against his skin would set off a whole new series of touching, retouching, and counting rituals. He needed to get to his dresser, get clean clothes, put them on, calculate the movements, memorize the order, do a mental rewind. It was exhausting, exasperating, and exhilarating to be clean again.

The water in the shower would be left running until Ed moved out of the shower and dressed, and only then could Michael move in and turn it off. It was a complex physical, and mental, dance that the two men did that day as Ed exposed himself, so to speak, to so many of the fears that haunted him. And as extraordinary an event as this was, Michael knew it was just one small step forward in Ed's treatment. But there were also the practical benefits of improved hygiene to consider—it would help in the healing of Ed's chronic bedsores, and Michael also hoped this step would lead to a new regimen of oral hygiene, the lack of which he feared was impacting Ed's general health.

Later that afternoon, Ed emerged from the basement to greet his waiting company. For a fleeting moment, he felt good about all that he'd accomplished, and hopeful. At the end of the visit, as wary as he was about having another new person infiltrate his space, he agreed to weekly visits with Lisa. But it was only because she was connected to Michael.

On the days Lisa was scheduled to visit, Tom or Tami would come to the house early in the morning and unlock the front door. For the first couple of visits, Ed made the extraordinary effort to come up from the basement and meet her upstairs in the living room. This was a three- to five-hour process of going up and down the stairs countless numbers of times until everything felt right. Once he was upstairs, he would sit on the edge of the sofa and patiently wait her arrival.

During the first few visits, Ed shared some of his drawings with Lisa. She encouraged his vision for having a future that involved getting back outside and finding work doing the thing he loved most, which, at this point, seemed to be the drawings. At one point, he actually acquiesced to a little bit of exposure therapy—when she asked him to try combing the short regrowth of hair on his head. But it was an incredibly painful experience for him as the bristles of the hairbrush touched his sensitive scalp. Immediately, and perhaps unsurprisingly, he obsessed over each individual bristle that touched his scalp, and he described the scratching noise with each brush as "nails to a chalkboard." "I tried," says Ed, "but it all happened too quick. I would be exhausted when she left, and my body shut down. It took me almost four hours to get upstairs, and back down, and it just wasn't worth it."

The novelty of Lisa's visits, having company in the middle of long, lonesome days, wore off quickly, and Ed stopped coming upstairs. When she arrived, she would walk down the steps leading to the basement where she would sit for hours and talk to Ed through the locked door. She would ask about his week and about new issues he might be struggling with, and she would take every opportunity to encourage him to reconsider coming back upstairs and trying behavioral therapy. But it was very clear that wasn't going to happen. "He's very, very intelligent, and he understood the *theory* behind the therapy, but we made very little progress in the actual practice of it," says Lisa. Ed actually thought behavioral therapy was nonsense.

In late summer of 1997, Ed's steadily increasing isolation became even more profound when he became desperately ill from food poisoning after he had eaten food that had been sitting out for two days.

Ed had no idea why he was consumed by violent nausea and vomiting. He was alone, barely able to make it to the bathroom, much less to the phone all the way down at the end of the hall. Ed was so sick he couldn't keep track of his movements or count the number of times he touched the floor with his hands as he tried to hold himself up. When he was finally able to crawl down the hall and call Tami, he pleaded for help because he was in so much pain. After she was able to calm him down a little bit, she implored him to hang up so she could drive over to the house and call Michael.

Michael, who talked Ed into calmly reenacting the events that led up to his feeling sick, concluded that he suffered from food poisoning. But the mental damage of having come so close to what he firmly believed was his own death was done. It was a terrifying episode. He replayed the scene over and over—reliving what it felt like to be sick, alone, *certain* that he was going to die. He thought about his mother, and he couldn't shake the image of her own passing from his mind. And to top it all off, he couldn't recapture all of the moments, and all of the movements he'd lost track of *while* he was sick. Time had progressed toward death in ways that he could no longer count.

Ed's clothes, the first set since he showered, were completely soiled with vomit, so he stripped them off, tied a black garbage bag around his waist like a kilt, and sat on the end of his bed, catatonic. His movements were limited to the daily trips to the basement door to collect the food that his sisters brought, although he ate very little of it. He lost weight, as he lived mostly on a diet of Gatorade. All of the Memorial Day shower hopefulness had been erased from his mind—not by his rituals, but by having been eclipsed by his physical illness.

And just when it seemed like things couldn't get worse, on one of the rare occasions that he looked out the basement window, he saw that the neighbors had torn down the stockade fence that separated the two properties and replaced it with a shorter one, altering the landscape of his basement perimeter. The world was changing, time was progressing, and Ed's mind was short-circuiting. Panic-stricken, he made the hours-long journey to the phone to call his neighbors at the time to explain his illness and the devastation replacing the fence caused him. Surprisingly, they agreed to let him replace the portion of the fence visible from the basement window.

So Ed called Walpole Woodworkers and talked to the manager, a guy named Carl Fister, telling him about what had happened; he explained his illness and the importance of rebuilding the section of fencing to look exactly as it had before it had been torn down. It had to be a "surgical operation," Ed told him because he could only replace that one specific section of fence and could not disturb the new, shorter fencing put in by the neighbors.

Carl agreed to come over to the house the next day to assess the work that had to be done. When he arrived, he sat patiently outside the basement door leading to the driveway, as Ed stood inside the doorway with only the black plastic bag around his waist. He told Ed it wasn't going to be easy to mesh the two different fences perfectly, but he would give it his best shot.

This had to be done perfectly, and Ed stood at the door three days later when Carl's team showed up to build the fence, wrapped in nothing but a garbage bag, ready to give instructions to the fence builders. He was the only one who knew exactly how it needed to look. Carl and his team, who understood how sick Ed actually was, were patient and kind.

As the fence was painstakingly reconstructed, a very compassionate Carl sat next to Ed, continuously reassuring him that his guys were going to make it right. He listened as Ed gave explicit directions about the height—or specific tilt—of the boards, took notes, and relayed those notes to his men. An hour and a half later, when the last plank was set, Carl turned to Ed to see if it was a job well done. Ed smiled, and for a fleeting moment, the anxiety dissipated, and he was momentarily safe.

**MICHAEL WOULD CONTINUE TRYING** to monitor Ed's progress by phone and visits to the Cape when his schedule permitted. By early 1998, Lisa had stopped her weekly visits, and Ed had tried every prescription medicine available for the treatment of OCD, without success. There was no hope that he would ever agree to come to the OCD Institute, and Michael, who admits to being emotionally invested at this point, was at a loss. "I felt like I'd tried everything," he recalls, "and despite the fact that I should be someone who knows how to get him out of there, I didn't really know what else to do. Ed's case was particularly poignant for me because we shared some kind of bond." Little did the all-but-defeated psychiatrist know that in the process of trying to treat Ed, he had planted a seed that was taking root deep down below all of the layers of mental anguish caused by Ed's OCD.

During a visit in March of 1998, with nothing left to offer from his vast experience and arsenal of traditional medicine and innovative therapy, Michael watched as a pitiful shadow of the Ed he first knew climbed the steps before him, arms outstretched like a zombie, trying to muster the best smile he could. It was one of the most profoundly sad and hopeless experiences of Michael's life. As he sat on the sofa in the Zine living room that day, Michael began to openly weep, wondering how, as sick as Ed was, he could manage a smile at all.

Ironically, it was Michael's tears of compassion that would touch Ed in such a way that it would change the course of his therapy, and his life.

# CHAPTER 13

# Forward in Time

◀◀

E D'S PAIN HAD BECOME MICHAEL'S sincere sorrow, and the compassion he had shown in that one vulnerable moment was a gift that would allow Ed to step outside of his condition and regain a certain perspective that had been lost. After Michael had run out of tears, the two spontaneously started laughing. "Through all of this, he could still smile and have a sense of humor about life," recalls Michael. But while Ed's sudden levity indicated a sudden revelation, Michael's signified resignation. He left that afternoon feeling defeated by the disorder he spent twenty years dissecting, consumed by his own inability to effect change in Ed's life. The two would remain in contact by phone, but it would be almost a year before they would meet again face-to-face.

During this time, Ed would not make any pronouncements about his new resolve. The blood of a prizefighter ran through his veins, and there was something in the way Michael dropped his guard that afternoon and wept for him that led the all-but-defeated patient to suddenly find his inner strength. That single moment provided a clarity for Ed that he'd never had before—OCD was the *enemy within him.*

"The day Dr. Jenike broke down in my living room, I was pissed off to holy hell and back," recalls Ed. "OCD was holding me back from living my life and being happy. It was hurting the people I cared about, and I wanted to kick the 'ever-loving' shit out of it."

It was a familiar rush of adrenaline and, like a hero ready to ride into battle and save the day, Ed positioned himself mentally to do battle against OCD. OCD would be his target, his enemy, and his singular focus. Using the full force of his enormous intellect, and perhaps some of the subconscious lessons of behavioral therapy his mind and body had openly rejected, he would defeat his enemy, and, in doing so, he would honor Michael and the people he loved. By finding a way to save himself, Ed would become the unwitting hero of his own life.

Using his analytical mind and the same meticulous thought processes that fueled his rituals—which were actually signs of not just illness, but uncanny genius—Ed determined that OCD had successfully amassed all of his fears, traumas, and weaknesses to form a formidable army of negative energy, and that what he needed to do to get control was to "flip the script."

OCD was the dark force that required Ed to do its bidding. Not only did the compulsions torment him, the impact it had on others created an enormous burden of guilt. By looking at it as the enemy, and visualizing OCD as an entity apart from himself, he could unwrap himself from that guilt and dissect its parts objectively. This created more space in his overburdened mind to *re*focus on making his greatest fear, not death, but an irrepressibly hopeless life.

Ed began to visualize OCD as a wall, once impenetrable, that had shown its first tiny crack. Michael made the first breakthrough when he planted a seed of trust by taking the time to get to know Ed as a person, not just a patient. And from years of working in construction with his father, Ed knew *every* wall had multiple unseen cracks—all he had to do now was to find them and exploit them for his benefit.

"I had to begin to force myself to drop all of my fears, and do just one thing at a time," says Ed. One step at a time may sound easy, but OCD sufferers struggle to compartmentalize tasks. For example, if someone without OCD has a list of ten things on a to-do list for the day, he or she can prioritize and move through each task one by one until the tasks are done. The person with OCD might look at the same list, obsess about the responsibility of all ten items at once, and become overwhelmed. "The brain goes into lockdown," says Ed. "That's why people get stuck, and when you get stuck, you feel like a failure." From there, depression can splinter off and mentally debilitate the OCD patient, thwarting any determination he or she has to get well, thus exacerbating the condition.

"It was like OCD was a bully in my head calling me a 'sucker,' and always saying, 'I don't think you can do that,'" says Ed. "I had to find a way to be one step ahead of my OCD at all times, and I needed a lot of praise and support to get me through it."

DESPITE ED'S NEW RESOLVE, HOWEVER, his need to stop the progression of time hadn't diminished, nor had his worries about keeping his family alive. His touching, counting, and checking rituals were still excessive. What *had* changed, however, was his focus and motivation to get well. He mentally sparred with OCD every waking minute, forcing himself to do fewer repetitions of his rituals. He began to draw more. OCD had never put constraints on his art, and he pushed himself to create complex images of people, and cartoon characters that he loved. But reaching out to friends and acquaintances *did* present a challenge.

"The phone rang," remembers Kevin Frye, Ed's old high school friend, "and when I picked it up, the operator said she had a call from Ed Zine. She said that he was very nervous about calling me because we hadn't spoken in a long time and asked me if I would please not hang up." It had been more than two years since Kevin had heard from Ed, and although he agreed to take the call, he thought it might be a prank call from one of his cousins known to make fun of Ed's quirky behavior from the days when Ed's symptoms first began to manifest themselves and he would take those seemingly odd detours on the way to McDonald's.

Kevin struggled to identify the weak, high-pitched voice on the other end of the phone. "It didn't sound anything like my cousin, or Eddie, but I kept the conversation going, trying to figure out who was playing the joke," says Kevin. As the conversation progressed, it soon became clear, as he began to share details of his illness and the visits from Dr. Jenike, that it was indeed the long-lost Ed Zine calling. Calling Kevin was an important first step for Ed in his efforts to recover because he didn't know how Kevin would react to the news of his illness. But he faced his fear, and Kevin's compassionate reaction was the reinforcement Ed needed to take *another* step forward.

**PART OF ED'S TREATMENT PLAN** for himself was to focus on the happiest moments of his life. This allowed him to get into an almost Zen-like state that gave him relief from his obsessive-compulsive behaviors for short bursts of time. The fact that most of his happiest memories occurred *before* his mother's death made it a challenge because the sadness of her death would inevitably disrupt the moment.

In an idea akin to the ancient Romans who built statues of their fallen heroes, Ed decided to memorialize his mother's life in a way that made the most sense to him. The best last memory of his mother was when Ed went to see *The Empire Strikes Back* shortly before her passing. And looking around at the *Star Wars* magazines piled on the floor, he began to believe that if he could acquire an original Darth Vader costume, it would help him honor that one important moment from his past, make him happy, and help him get on the path to recovery. It would be his link to the days when his mother sat in the kitchen at the table as he traipsed around the house in his Darth Vader costume playing *Star Wars*. This became the happy thought that consumed him.

Don Post, head of the world-renowned Don Post Studios, which held one of the first licensing agreements with Lucas Films for *Star Wars* helmets and life-sized replicas, wasn't in his office the first time Ed made the long trek across the basement to try and reach him by phone. A celebrity to *Star Wars* fans around the world, Don has a deep appreciation for the people who value his work, and he makes a conscious effort to respond to the fans who reach out to him; but trying to speak individually to the thousands of people who have contacted him in the twenty-five years since the film first premiered, simply to talk about all things *Star Wars*, is impossible. He rarely answers the phone himself, and it is unusual for fans to get past the secretary.

As it turned out, Don's youngest son, Josh, was fielding phone calls at the office the day Ed called. A skilled and compassionate listener who holds a degree in youth and family ministries, Josh listened carefully as Ed told him the story of his mother's death, his OCD, and how he believed that acquiring a Darth Vader costume would help him honor his mother and emphasize the happier times in his life so he could heal and begin to live again. Josh had actually studied OCD in school while getting his degree, and he had a modest understanding of the disorder and at least an appreciation for its degrees of severity.

"What stood out to me," remembers Josh, "was that he was a very nice, loving person who was tragically trapped in this disease, and I felt very sorry for him."

Initially, Ed had no idea that he was speaking to Don's son—Josh didn't immediately identify his relationship—but he knew that, whomever the speaker was, he clearly had access to Don. Ed spoke frantically, not wanting Josh to hang up before he could tell his entire story. He repeated himself over and over, nervously wanting to get all of the details right. "I got off the phone and I felt exhausted from talking in circles," says Josh, who eventually revealed his identity and agreed to have his father return Ed's call. For the thirty minutes after they hung up, Ed, excited and happy, sat by the phone and waited as he replayed their conversation backward and forward until the phone rang again.

**DON POST IS A KIND, SOFT-SPOKEN** Christian man who sincerely believes that everyone has some sort of calling and that *his* is to minister to the people who come into his life and need his help. He doesn't necessarily feel obligated to go seeking people in need, but he says when God sends someone to his doorstep, he makes himself available. So, when Josh tracked him down on the manufacturing floor and told him Ed's story, there was no question Don felt he was being called into service.

As excited as Ed was when the phone finally rang—he instinctively knew it was Don calling—he waited for an even number of rings before picking up. For the next hour and a half, he anxiously recounted his story, not only talking about the loss of his mother and the significance of *The Empire Strikes Back,* but also sharing intricate details of his life in isolation, his commitment to Pembroke Hospital, and the help Dr. Jenike had tried to give him. Periodically, Ed would, per usual, repeat sentences and words to satisfy his anxiety and even drop out of the conversation for several seconds so he could address his counting rituals. Despite his compulsions, however, his objective was clear—to convince Don Post to help him acquire a life-sized Darth Vader costume.

Don remembers, "He was a very thoughtful and gentle person, but it was like trying to communicate in the middle of a tornado." Not only was it hard to sort through Ed's repetition of thoughts and ideas, but also "It was so difficult and grueling to hear what he'd gone through." Don explained to Ed that he no longer had a license to make a full Darth Vader costume and wasn't sure what he could do to help, but that he would give some thought to other options Ed might explore. Despite the realities of what it would take to acquire this costume, Ed hung up the phone filled with hope, and he believed that somehow Don would find a way to help him make this need in his life a reality. At the end of the conversation, Ed asked Don if he would call back again, explaining the compulsive need for him to call twice. Don obliged.

Don's intense conversation with Ed left him with a headache that lasted for a full two days, but he couldn't stop thinking about the situation, and he wanted to find a way to help Ed. He knew this was about more than placating an obsessed fan. It was about saving a life. So Don says he called in a favor to Steve Sansweet, the director of content management and head of fan relations at Lucas Films, who also happens to own the largest private collection of *Star Wars* memorabilia in the world and has written several books on the subject. In a completely unprecedented move, Don says Steve agreed to help him get the special permissions he needed to make one replica. Don then solicited the help of friends in the business to produce it at cost, and he offered his own time and materials, gratis, to get the job done.

**ED WANTED TO DO SOMETHING** to show his gratitude for the kindness Josh had shown in getting his father on the phone and decided to send him some of his artwork to Los Angeles, but he didn't have the postage or packaging. So he called the post office to see if someone could drop off the supplies he needed. It wasn't typical protocol, and the only person who could make that call was Cape Cod Postmaster Peter Mackiewicz. Peter had heard about Ed from one of the carriers who delivered mail to his house. He didn't know what his illness was, but if this desperate man needed help, Peter wanted to be part of the solution. After all, he'd made a promise.

PETER WOULD NEVER FORGET STANDING in the hallway of Massachusetts General Hospital and making that deal with God. If He would only save his five-year-old son, he would spend the rest of his days in His service. The prognosis for the little boy's cancer was grim, and doctors wanted to try cranial radiation—a procedure that had previously had a very low success rate and often resulted in mental retardation. But the situation was desperate, and because of refinements in the way the radiation was targeted, the doctors hoped for a more successful outcome.

Peter got the miracle he prayed for that day; his son would grow up cancer free. But he would never forget the promise he made to God and vowed to help anyone in need. And then Ed came into his life.

Peter told Ed exactly what time he'd be arriving to drop off the packing supplies.

Ed told him to wait in the driveway, and as Ed made his way, tentatively, up the side steps from the basement toward the mail truck, Peter remembers, "It was frightening. He was thin, malnourished, and hunched over like an old man. His hair was standing straight up, and he was unshaven." Little did Peter realize at the time that Ed had just climbed a mountain.

After the two met and spoke for a few minutes, Ed paid for his supplies, and Peter gave Ed his number and told him that if he needed anything else from the post office, he should just call him directly. Then Peter watched in amazement as Ed walked backward up the driveway, about twenty feet, and backward down the steps—carefully placing his feet in exactly the same places he had walked to get there—then disappeared backward through the door. "I thought this poor kid must really be crazy," says Peter.

That night, Peter told his wife exactly what he'd seen, and he wondered what kind of mental illness would make someone act that way. Whatever it was, he knew he needed to see Ed again to find out more.

Ed's correspondence with Don Post via mail became more frequent as the efforts to design the life-size Darth Vader costume progressed. He used the number Peter had given him to call and ask for assistance whenever he had packages to send, and Peter used this opportunity to get to know Ed better, often volunteering to come over and pick up the packages himself. In time, Ed shared the details of his illness, the story of Darth Vader, and his relationship with Don Post. Peter didn't understand obsessive-compulsive disorder, or how it *should* be treated, but as a longtime Little League coach, he understood the importance of overcoming little hurdles to reach big plateaus; and although he wasn't a doctor, he felt he could use this approach to help inspire Ed to take little steps that would lead him to the bigger life that he desired.

**AS MUCH AS ED APPRECIATED** Don Post's efforts, there was mounting frustration over the details of the Darth Vader replica that was being designed in Los Angeles. Not only did Ed possess a photographic memory, he had seen *The Empire Strikes Back* at least a thousand times and his OCD demanded that the replica be absolutely perfect, matching exactly what was in his mind. Unfortunately, the photographs, drawings, paint, and material samples that went back and forth in the mail between L.A. and Cape Cod, were not, according to Ed, an exact match.

Of course Don knew it was impossible for two hand-constructed Darth Vader costumes to ever be *perfectly* alike, but he felt he'd come as close as was humanly possible to making Ed's replica perfect. Don knew Ed was sick, and a letter from Dr. Jenike had validated the facts; still, he was taken aback at the intensity of the demands OCD placed upon Ed. In one instance, Don shared what he thought was very good news, proudly telling Ed that he was able to secure a piece of the exact material used in the grid of the mask and that he had the original Chrysler Corporation paint colors that were used on the helmet, which in the movie appears to be black but, in actuality, is a mix of black and silver paint to give the original helmet a greater dimension during filming. But when he sent the sample via mail, Ed rejected both specs, saying they were wrong and did not match the Vader he saw in the movie.

The last thing in the world that Ed wanted was to be difficult, but he had this uncontrollable need for perfection—well, that *and* the premier mask manufacturer in the world. "The reality is I've seen and touched the original thing," says Don, "and there is a very specific kind of grid in the original helmet, and I had acquired a piece of it, but Ed's *impression* of what he'd seen on the screen—and he'd watched *Empire Strikes Back* more than a thousand times—was different, and he swore it wasn't the right stuff." Don said as much as he knew about Darth Vader, Ed actually knew more.

The discussions over the phone between Ed and Don were difficult. Don was doing what he does best but was being told it wasn't right; Ed's OCD demanded that he have exactly what he needed in order to get well. "Imagine standing on the bow of a ship in the middle of a blizzard, and trying to carry on a conversation," says Don, trying to assess the difficulty in speaking with

Ed. "That's how trying our discussions were." Before long, they were at an impasse "I knew it was his OCD demanding these things," says Don, "but I also knew whatever I did would never be good enough." Ultimately, as much sympathy as he had for Ed's situation, Don refused to continue constructing the Darth Vader replica.

"I told him I was done with it," says Don. "'I'll be your friend, but I don't want to talk about *Star Wars* and Darth Vader anymore.'" It wasn't an easy conversation for Don to have after several months of working together to try and get this right, and of course it was a terrible disappointment for Ed.

Still, the two would continue to talk periodically over the phone, and they would remain friends as Ed continued his search for the "perfect" life-sized replica of Darth Vader. Ed says the reason that he was not satisfied with the Darth Vader Don Post was trying to make was not because of OCD or being difficult—that it was the Darth Vader from *Star Wars: A New Hope*, not *The Empire Strikes Back*.

But Ed persisted and says he eventually acquired a "screen-used" complete Darth Vader costume from *The Empire Strikes Back* and a touring suit from London, which he claims was confirmed as authentic by Steve Sansweet.

IN THE MEANTIME, PETER MACKIEWICZ continued to stop by the house and check on Ed to see how he was doing. Each time they spoke, Peter became bolder in his efforts to encourage Ed to step out of his safety zone and try new things. "I told him he needed to get cleaned up, showered, and eat something," says Peter. "He looked like he was starving." Ed explained to Peter that while his family stopped by with food once a day, it was too hard to go up and down the stairs to the kitchen any other time, even if he *was* still hungry, because the rewinding and repeating—the number of times that often took him into five digits—were just too exhausting.

Peter pushed him, "Why so many, Ed? Why not do just twenty-five times?" Ed told him that would never work because he had to do it an even number of times. Then he asked Peter if he could repeat a process ten times. "Why not?" encouraged Peter, who wasn't aware he was encouraging the kind of behavioral therapy that Ed needed to do to continue getting better.

Every day, Ed continued to remind himself that OCD was his enemy. He was at war, and the battle was to try and limit the number of times he counted, checked, and reversed his actions. By October of 1998, he had pushed the boundaries of his OCD world beyond the basement and into the driveway, where he would often meet Peter to talk. He soon surprised his brother, Tom, when, for the first time in more than two years, he asked if they could go for a ride in the car. "I wanted to show everyone that I was really trying to make strides to get better," says Ed.

Tom took Ed on a routine errand to the CVS Pharmacy at the Cape Cod Mall in Hyannis, careful to avoid rotaries and the left-hand turns that he knew would aggravate Ed's OCD. But it was still a terrifying twenty-mile journey for Ed. The minute they arrived, Ed got out of the car and began walking forward and backward, over and over, in front of the building, trying to find relief from the anxiety of the drive and having left the house. While Tom ran inside the store, a middle-aged man who'd been watching Ed retrace his steps walked by and remarked in a loud voice, "What a fucking retard."

Ed was crushed. It was a brutal comment that brought a devastating end to a trip that started out with so much hope for progress. All the way home, he sat in the car seat rocking back and forth, counting higher and higher in even numbers of multiples, rewinding the trip in his mind, talking backward to himself. Tom gave Ed comfort and support, telling him, "It's going to be okay, brother, it's going to be okay," until they were able to get home and get Dr. Jenike on the phone.

This was the first time that Michael got wind of any of Ed's progress. They'd spoken on the phone, but Ed kept his efforts to himself in the hope that when he got well, he would surprise Michael with his recovery. The anticipation of this moment was one of the things that motivated Ed to keep trying harder. Michael was at once amazed at Ed's big step and concerned. He had to respond quickly to Ed's experience at CVS to help him avoid a total setback. "It's *his* inability to take the time to understand you first," Michael told Ed, who was still reeling. "It's *his* ignorance." The logic with which Michael assessed the situation actually hit home with Ed. He had just "flipped the script" and allowed Ed to actually conclude that, "It was not me, it was him."

Even during this conversation, Ed didn't explain to Michael how he now approached OCD as his enemy, and the strides he was making outside this attempt to escape the basement. He wanted to save everything else for the moment he had planned in his head—the picture-perfect movie ending when he would walk out of the basement and show Michael that he had worked hard to honor everything he'd done for him. He wasn't going to spoil that moment by giving it away in pieces too soon.

Coming out of the basement, and trying to integrate himself into the outside world while having to fulfill the demands of

OCD was precarious, but Ed wanted it so badly. He wasn't going to let the cruelty of an idiot stranger at CVS stop him, but he would look for a place to go where he wouldn't be judged harshly and he could avoid gawking strangers on the street. So, shortly after the CVS experience, he called a taxi, climbed in, and took a ride to his friend Kevin's house.

Ed didn't know what to expect, and he didn't know if he'd have the courage to go through with it, so he made the visit unannounced. When he arrived in front of Kevin's house, he asked the cab driver to wait by the curbside in case Kevin wasn't home. When Kevin's wife answered the door and told Ed that he wasn't home, Ed quietly thanked her and proceeded to walk backward all the way down the sidewalk and climb backward into the cab. Even though Kevin was unavailable, Ed had successfully exposed himself to the fear of going out, alone, and the ride was not as terrifying as he'd imagined it would be. It was a building block for success.

Although OCD continued to make incessant demands of Ed, his confidence was building. He was enjoying the incremental freedom, the kind the unafflicted take for granted, as he pushed back the boundaries of his isolation. As the winter unfolded, Ed was taking more car rides with his family and generally getting out of the house more often. The basement was still his safe haven, he still struggled with hygiene, he still counted and retraced his steps and refused to walk on the cracks of tile, but at least he was getting outside.

One day, Ed suggested to Peter that he might actually like to try driving on his own. Privately, Peter was nervous as he thought about the importance of "little hurdles," and he was worried that Ed might be trying too much too soon.

But in February of 1999, Ed called Diamond Chevrolet in Worcester, Massachusetts, where his uncle Duddie and cousin David Massad worked. He told them about his OCD and explained that he needed a certain type of vehicle that wouldn't make him feel like he was in a coffin. His best option was an SUV, and they did everything in their power to accommodate him. They settled on an Eddie Bauer Ford Expedition, and all the paperwork was done by them, because it was too hard for Ed to read a lengthy contract back and forth hundreds of times. They even delivered the car to his front door. When they showed up it represented more than a car to Ed. It represented freedom from OCD's prison. Ed says the first time he drove his new car, he felt like he was Charlton Heston riding a chariot in *Ben Hur*.

Tom, Tami, and Deena were cautiously optimistic about the progress Ed was making, but they, too, worried that he might be moving too fast. However, they also didn't want to discourage him, and they did what they could to help Ed from the moment he made plans to purchase a new car. During this time, no one called Michael to clue him in about what was happening, but when *he* called to check in, Ed would talk about family and sports—everything but his progress.

Two months later, to Peter's utter surprise, Ed showed up at the post office driving a brand-new car. But not everything went perfectly. Peter recalls, "Even with the car, Ed was still self-conscious about going out in public—his hygiene was still not great, and he wore the same clothes all the time." And having a new car didn't erase Ed's anxiety about the way he looked and how strangers would respond to him. He expectedly struggled with driving in certain directions and had to avoid rotaries and medians in the middle of the road that felt "bad." Peter encouraged him to focus on taking small trips, starting with the post office. He told Ed to call before he left the house and that he would always be on the lookout for his arrival.

*Entering* the post office was a big ordeal for Ed—he was embarrassed about the way he looked and acted. But knowing Peter was there waiting for him gave him the courage he needed to try. He would enter the lobby sideways, with the back heel of his foot going through the entrance first. Then he would spin around the other way quickly to give the appearance of walking in normally. In actuality, he had entered the lobby backward and, when he left, he would walk out normally, completing the cycle.

One day, a few weeks after Ed first got his car, he showed up in the lobby, and Peter couldn't believe his eyes. "He was clean, he had on a new set of clothes, he'd shaved, and he looked like an all-American kid—the change was remarkable." Peter suggested that Ed drive down to the oceanfront and just sit in the parking lot and relax where no one could see him if he felt the need to get out of the car and walk backward. Just being out, Peter felt, was enough of an accomplishment.

As soon as Ed bought his car, he started thinking about how to make his way back to the gym. On his first day back, he felt like it was 1992 all over again—and 1992 was a good year. None of the old guys were there—it was a completely new crew—and he put his heart and soul into getting in good physical condition.

By May of 1999, Ed was getting out of the house on a regular basis. He was driving to his sister's house, eating out at McDonald's, and drawing more regularly. He'd even returned to his routine at the gym. And he was ready to show Michael how far he'd come, and the true meaning of honor.

# CHAPTER 14

# Time Changes Everything

◀◀

WHEN MICHAEL PULLED SHUT THE front door of Ed's house in Cape Cod after their emotional meeting in March of 1998, he didn't expect to come back anytime soon. Ed had given him an air hug—the pantomime act of reaching his arms around Michael without touching him—to say good-bye. There was nothing more, medically, that Michael felt he could offer. He resigned himself to the idea that Ed would most likely spend the rest of his life living in his father's basement unless he became able to leave the house and agreed to submit himself to residential treatment. Michael now had to focus on his research and the patients he *could* help. He would stay in touch, he told Ed, and for the next year he was true to his word, but the two spoke only by phone.

Filled with emotion, and a deep sense of loss, Michael pulled out of the driveway and made his way a few miles closer to Boston before steering his car to the side of the road and breaking down.

Ed says he didn't feel abandoned, because he knew Michael would keep his word and stay in touch, but he also knew, instinctively, that Michael wouldn't be back to see him anytime soon. But this last meeting was a turning point—it was the first time he'd been witness to this kind of a display of emotion—a visible demonstration of sheer compassion and concern. Regardless of how much his family cared about him, and they *did* care, since their mother's death everyone had pushed through his or her pain with a "stiff upper lip," holding in their feelings and emotions.

Ed became angry when the door closed that day—not at Michael for leaving, but angry at the OCD—the thief that had stolen so much of his life and pushed away the people he cared about. Being pissed off at OCD allowed Ed to recapture his determination and spirit. This experience was his wake-up call.

Ed looked up to Michael like a big brother, but regardless of how affable and down-to-earth Michael was when he came to visit, it never escaped Ed that Michael was a world-class physician who drove the six-hour round-trip to care for him, armed with compassion and wanting absolutely nothing in return. And when all that failed, he generously offered his friendship. In Ed's world, that meant he *owed* Michael something—semper fidelis— always faithful. They had served in this battle together, and he would keep fighting OCD and find a way to honor the sacrifices Michael had made for him.

During every victory, from making the call to Don Post, to climbing each cement step up the side of the house to meet Peter,

Ed played a movie scene in his head—the moment he would walk out of the house into the sunshine happy, healthy, and fit, ready to surprise Michael.

**WHEN MICHAEL AND ED SPOKE** on the phone, the conversations were usually pretty casual, having little to do with OCD. Michael would occasionally suggest another attempt at cognitive behavioral therapy or float the idea of Ed coming to the OCD Institute, but Ed never took the bait.

Ed was very strategic in how little information he shared with Michael, not wanting to give away too much and spoil the surprise scene he had created in his mind. Michael knew Ed was trying to make some progress, and that he had *tried* the car trip to CVS with Tommy because, of course, he had to help Ed cope with the repercussions of that trip, but he didn't know the outings continued. He knew about the calls to Don Post because Ed asked him to write the letter confirming his OCD, but he didn't know about the friendship he formed with Peter. So Michael had no gauge of how well Ed was managing his OCD when he drove to the Cape the following spring.

It was an extraordinary spring day in May of 1999 when Michael took the three-hour drive to the Cape. Michael may have noticed there was *something* different in the tone of Ed's voice when they talked in the days leading up to his visit—a quiet strength that hadn't been there before—but he had no reason to think this visit would be different from the rest when a frail Ed Zine would ascend the steps from the basement to the living room to greet him.

When Michael pulled his sports car in front of the house

and turned off the engine, he saw a big guy standing in the driveway next to a new Ford Expedition. He was a good-looking young man—tanned, clean-cut, and looking like a cross between a professional football player and a marine. Michael didn't have any idea who he was—Ed hadn't mentioned having company—so when he walked up the driveway, he reached out his hand and introduced himself.

Ed flashed a brilliant, white smile, grabbed Michael's hand, and wrapped his big arms around him, laughing. Michael, not easily shocked, was completely flabbergasted. How was this possible? All he could manage to say was, "What have you done with *my* Ed?"

The moment was everything Ed had imagined and hoped it would be—the fact that Michael hadn't recognized him was a perfectly executed scene—it couldn't have been written any better. The two men stood back and looked at each other—Ed almost giddy at the shock on Michael's face, and Michael holding back the tears as his mind tried to reconcile the sight of the man who stood before him with his memory of the sad, frail Ed crippled by OCD that he'd last seen.

Some would call it a miracle, but Michael was a scientist, and questions immediately began pounding his brain . . . *how, what, why, and when* . . . he had to know.

There were so many things that Ed had planned to say to Michael. He wanted to tell him how their last visit had allowed him to flip the script and that OCD was his enemy; how hard he fought to stop the thousands of repetitive movements; how much he wanted to live a "normal" life; and how he did all of this not only to honor himself but also to honor Michael's sacrifice of time. But Ed's mind was moving at lightning speed, and his anxiety was rising. Ed's OCD wasn't *gone,* it was just being *managed*—he wanted to explain this, too. But before he got "stuck" and derailed in the crashing of thoughts, he needed to focus and move on to the next step of his plan.

"I'm hungry," said Ed. "Do you want to go get something to eat?" This casual suggestion was another in a series of incomprehensible developments that day, but it was followed by an even bigger surprise after Michael agreed. "Okay," said Ed, "I'll drive."

In the car, as Ed tried to hold back the waves of checking and counting rituals that overwhelmed him, he talked in circles, trying to explain to Michael what had happened, as he tried desperately to keep track of the words and phrases he was using for the mental rewind later that day. It was an emotionally charged monologue filled with a message of gratitude. He talked about how honor was his bond with Michael, and that's what helped him heal, and he gushed about Michael being his hero and his brother. But at that moment, none of it was registering with Michael because his scientific brain was spinning in high gear, and he wanted to know the process that had brought Ed to this incredible place in his management of OCD. He needed to know exactly how this happened so he could figure out how to apply this experience and help the other desperately ill patients who needed their miracles, too. But everything Ed said about *how* he got better was emotional—it did not connect to Michael's logic.

Although there are countless OCD patients who look at Michael as something of a hero, it is not a comfortable notion for him. Life has taught him, in the cruelest of ways, an appreciation for its brevity, and he has a sense of urgency to use his time on earth to ease the suffering of human beings. He doesn't see that as heroism, he sees it as the obligation of every human being.

He is an intelligent, sensitive, and often shy man, with a twisted sense of humor who much prefers to spend his days flying under everyone's radar, playing basketball every chance he gets, and solving problems. Accolades and ego are not what drive him.

"Michael has a hard time giving up on people," says Diane Davey, the program manager and director of administration for the OCD Institute, "especially when everybody else has already said, 'I can't help.'" The "Leave no man or woman behind" philosophy is part of the makeup that compels Michael to advocate for those patients in the most extreme situations, offering hope for management of their symptoms when others have deemed them untreatable. Ed was not the first among them.

In the population of patients suffering from OCD for whom Michael has fought, there are other extraordinary stories of housebound victims living their lives in a tangle of rituals and uncontrollable thoughts, like the woman who washed her hands more than twelve hours a day, for fifteen years, in a series of extreme, complicated rituals, using bleach. One patient, a gentle young man diagnosed with terminal cancer sought treatment for intrusive thoughts, all unfounded, that he might sexually molest a child or harm someone. The pain of his obsessions was so insufferable that he told Michael if he were given the option to cure his unrelenting OCD or his terminal cancer, he would choose to eradicate the OCD. These are the people who define the very essence of what OCD means to Michael, and he is only too aware of the fact that too many stay hidden in their secret worlds of shame, lacking awareness and understanding of their behavior, while only the fortunate among them eventually find their way to treatment and support.

Michael understood that Ed had all of these ideas about honoring the people he cares about. He knew that Ed didn't like to disappointment people and that if he makes a commitment, he is compelled to keep it. But Ed never made a commitment to him to get better. He never actually said those words to Michael. So Ed's resolve *and* results confirmed what Michael had always suspected—that in the treatment of cancer or any other disorder, the relationship between the patient and physician is a very important component. And in Ed's case, it seemed it was the most important part of what helped Ed move forward. Indeed, the human relationship aspect was critical. But where was the science?

At the end of the day, Ed tapped into his extraordinary genius to unlock his own mind, subconsciously, applying bits of theory he'd been taught by Lisa and developing his own tenacious, customized version of exposure and response therapy. Inspired by Michael, he found a way to manage his OCD on his own through cognitive therapy techniques. It would take several years for Michael and Ed to fully understand how Ed got himself out of the basement. Now, it was time for Ed to move on to the next act of his movie. The first was tragic, the second was transformative, and this, the third, would be all about the girl.

# CHAPTER 15

# Mayada

⏪

**E**D **SILENTLY COUNTED HIS STEPS** as he headed down the gently sloped sidewalk of the Landfall Restaurant in Woods Hole, Massachusetts. The sky above him was seaside blue with pearls of white mist breaking across the sun as seagulls all around him stretched their wings to the rhythm of their slow, undulating cries. In the distance, Ed could hear the sounds of the steamship authority ferry going to Martha's Vineyard, and the rolling waves of the midday ocean as its brackish scent permeated the air.

For anyone watching from the outside patio, there were no signs of OCD's past torture. And while Ed wasn't *cured*, because there is no "cure" for OCD, he had traveled a million miles from his horrific life in the basement and was managing his OCD in a way that allowed him to go out for lunch and enjoy this beautiful Cape Cod day in May of 1999.

As Ed entered the crowded restaurant, he made his way around tables of strangers, counting and remembering the location of each chair and making a mental note of each maneuver so he could reverse the trek on his way out of the restaurant. Ed would always have to manage the constant drumbeat of obsessive thoughts that tapped in his brain, but his ability to "manage" his OCD meant that he would modify its demands. If his OCD *demanded* he walk around a chair twelve times to feel okay, he would negotiate a lesser number in his mind. Managing OCD was a constant struggle, but as he continuously exposed himself to the anxiety of doing fewer repetitions for any given action, his anxiety level would decrease. He had brilliantly figured out a way to practice classic exposure and response therapy without even knowing it.

But Ed's integration into some semblance of a "normal" life was exhausting. Going to the gym, for example, was a half-day project. It would often take him thirty or forty minutes just to get out the door of the house and into the car as he fought back the OCD desire to meticulously repeat and rewind his actions. His life was a continuous mental negotiation with his OCD.

SITTING WITH FRIENDS THAT DAY at the Landfall Restaurant was a young woman named Mayada, who looked up and saw Ed walking down the sidewalk. Mayada was one of six children born to an American nurse and a Palestinian pharmacist who met while they were in college. After her parents' divorce, she'd lived in Palestine with her father, a warm and gentle man, until the age of thirteen, and she had been living back in the States for nine years.

Ed had not come to the restaurant to meet anyone in particular; he had simply come to have lunch and get out of the house that had held him captive for so long. But he'd made a critical decision as he forced himself out of isolation. He would not be ashamed of his life, his OCD, and the frightening way in which he lived. "What got me out of the basement was being able to finally admit who I am. I decided not to judge myself, but to just be me." Whenever the opportunity presented itself, Ed would talk openly about his experience with OCD.

Individuals with OCD do judge themselves, and their illogical behavior, more harshly than any outside observer ever could, because they *know* it doesn't make any sense, and they *hate* the way their mind thinks and forces them to act. Ed's ability to come to terms with this was crucial in his progression to a manageable phase.

The Landfall Restaurant is a popular gathering place for locals, and when Ed arrived, he ran into some acquaintances and sat down to talk. The conversation soon turned to Ed's experience with OCD.

Mayada had not taken her eyes off Ed as he entered the restaurant and crossed the floor to take a seat with his friends at the table next to her. "It may sound crazy," she says, "but when I saw him, all the music stopped, everything got quiet, and everything stood perfectly still. It was *truly* love at first sight.

"In the Palestinian world," says Mayada, "mental illness was viewed as something shameful. The afflicted were kept behind closed doors." But although she had little experience with people with debilitating mental illness, let alone the type of OCD Ed was suffering, she had a natural compassion for this man on whom she was eavesdropping as he shared his difficult tale with their common friends.

Mayada knew some of the people sitting at Ed's table, and as chairs emptied over the next hour, she moved to get closer to Ed, and she became involved in the conversation. "There was something so special about him," she recalls. "He was not your average muscle guy. He was so gentle, and polite." By the time Ed was ready to leave, Mayada had made her way to the chair next to his, and as he started to get up from the table, she gently reached over, put her hand on his knee, and asked him not to go.

Ed had not been touched like that in years, but while that sort of spontaneous reaction could have just *weeks* before created enormous anxiety, there was something familiar and warm about this woman. The fact that Mayada was a beautiful woman didn't escape Ed. But this wasn't a sensual touch—it was, more important, a *loving* touch. Surprised that she would want to hear more about his life, he smiled and sat back down. He found himself easily sharing the more difficult and grueling details of his disrupted life, wanting to communicate it all to her so she would know exactly who he was. Mayada recalls that before the night was over, he told her he was looking for "someone to hold the other half of his heart in her hand."

As shocking as it may have been for Mayada to hear that the man who had just swept her off her feet suffered from severe OCD, had been committed to a psychiatric hospital, and had recently emerged from almost three years locked in a basement, she was unwavering in her compassion and awe. "Ed was amazing; he had come through all of this on his own, and nothing he said to me changed the way I felt from the first minute I saw him." And even though she knew nothing of OCD, Ed sensed in Mayada a girl who could be his best friend and someone who would reach out a hand to pick him up if he fell—the kind of girl he would have been proud to take home to his mother. He felt her father's greatness of heart, and her mother's compassion as a nurse. At the end of the evening, after hours of talking, the two exchanged phone numbers.

IN THE WEEK FOLLOWING HIS meeting with Mayada, he thought about her often, but the idea of actually calling her was nerve-racking. Ed worried that his OCD would require him to call multiple times and that she might think he was a stalker. On the other end of town, Mayada was losing patience *waiting* for him to make that call.

IN SPITE OF ALL THE progress he'd made, the basement was still Ed's safety net—the comfortable retreat to which he escaped at the end of his daily struggle to manage his OCD. Surprisingly, though, he no longer faced his father's wrath. Bob had come a long way in his understanding of Ed's disorder since Michael Jenike entered the picture, and the father and son had slowly begun to repair their relationship. Dad was proud of how far Ed had come, and he desperately hoped nothing would stop his progress.

On the day Mayada first called, Bob was at the house and picked up the phone. When he heard a woman's voice on the line asking for Ed, he immediately felt protective—he wanted to know her intentions and didn't hesitate to ask. Mayada gently explained that she wanted to invite Ed to go Rollerblading. Assuaged by her friendly demeanor and open appreciation for Ed's condition, he handed the phone over to Ed, leaving her by saying simply, "Be gentle with my boy, he's been through a lot."

Ed's nervousness about going on his first date in more than five years was compounded by the fact that he'd never been on skates before, and the fact that he worried he might fall and hurt her. But Mayada was a skilled Rollerblader, and as she glided along the bike path next to him, she carefully monitored Ed's progress, knowing this was a very big step for him, concerned that he was comfortable. As Ed looked at the lithe woman who slipped her hand into his as he steadied himself on his skates, it was all the reassurance he needed that day.

The trust between Ed and Mayada was, quite inexplicably, a foregone conclusion, and the relationship developed quickly. She was soon dropping by Ed's house, unannounced, to visit, and making him tuna fish sandwiches and lemonade for lunch. As incredulous as it seems, she loved him wholly and unconditionally, and it was exactly the kind of love he needed to find the courage to walk her down the stairs and into the basement of his father's home where the remnants of his old life lay perfectly in place. If there was a "test" of true love—it was this.

It was a dark, haunted museum, cluttered with the carefully hoarded memories of his old life. Everything remained situated in its perfect place—suspended in time. The Ziploc bags and Gatorade bottles were gone, but the rings where they had sat for so long around the bed had left permanent stains on the floor, leaving an indelible mark of the time that had bound him. In the weeks following their first date, Mayada would spend a lot of time among the chaos, sitting next to Ed on the edge of the bed, holding his hand, and doing what he loved most—watching movies on television.

It certainly wasn't easy for Ed to allow Mayada into the part of his world that OCD still had such a strong hold on, and it provoked tremendous anxiety as she moved about the room, but he loved having her around and desperately fought the urge to avoid having her there. Mayada was sensitive to Ed's OCD—constantly asking questions with every move, trying to understand how her actions would impact him. And as much as she *wanted* to simply clean the basement for him, and it certainly would have been more comfortable for her if she had, she understood clearly that it wouldn't help him.

"I knew who Ed was as a person. He was a good man, and a strong man, and when he was ready, I knew he could fix it, so it didn't matter to me," says Mayada, who made a vow to herself that *she* would give Ed the support she knew he so desperately needed, because she felt no one had ever really been there for Ed consistently during his life, particularly during his childhood after his mother's death.

As unimaginable as it is to think that Mayada could tolerate the disorganization in which Ed still lived—yes, the dirty old comforter still lay across his bed, the odors still lingered, and everything had to stay in its proper place—it is the laughter they shared in spite of the environment that she remembers most. "We'd go upstairs and make dinner together, and then we'd stay up late playing all the old video games. Donkey Kong was our favorite."

Once, during their early days of dating, Ed recalled a day in 1992—a very good year in his life and a year that, when repeated verbally, is actually a trigger to help him calm down when his anxiety soars—when he, Tom, and a couple friends were sitting at a TCBY counter, enjoying banana splits after spending the better part of the afternoon at a driving range in Falmouth.

While there, Ed looked up and noticed the girl behind the counter serving ice cream who was staring at him and smiling— she was a pretty girl with long curly hair and a cute little gap in her front teeth, about sixteen years old, and he remembers thinking to himself, *She's checking me out.*

Before Ed asked the question, he already knew the answer.

"Are you the girl from TCBY?"

Mayada answered, "Yes." It was kismet.

What Ed remembers most in those early days is the gentleness he recognized as so similar to his mother's. Ed lost the first great love of his life at such a young age, and now, incredibly, his fractured life with OCD did not disqualify him from finding that same unconditional love again.

THE DETAILS OF THEIR GROWING intimacy and how it was impacted by Ed's OCD is something the couple will not discuss, but—without question—the couple "managed" the situation to their great satisfaction.

One morning, as Mayada was preparing to leave for work at a local department store, Ed leaned over, put his hands on her waist, and gave her a gentle kiss on the lips. Without saying a word, he gave her a second kiss to make it an even number and realized it was time to flip the script again. In order to make their relationship work the way he wanted it to, he had to make a choice—his OCD or the beautiful woman in his arms.

When she was gone, Ed stood in front of the *Running Man* laser disc for more than an hour, contemplating whether or not he should throw it away. His logical mind *knew* that this was the next big step in taking back his life and his future. But his OCD, which comprised his *illogical* mind, tried to convince him that something awful might happen to her should he move that disc. His anxiety soared, his heart raced, the nails screeched down the chalkboard, and his head spun. The burden was unbearable.

To calm himself down, Ed began to visualize a daisy and the pulling of each petal as he whispered, "She loves me, she loves me not, she loves me, she loves me not, she loves me. . . ." And on the last "she loves me," he took a deep breath, picked up *Running Man*, reached for a green trash bag—like the ones he used to wear around his waist—and threw it inside. He talked himself through every move, "don't stop, keep moving, don't stop, keep moving," as he grabbed the dog shampoo that belonged to Zeus that had sat on top of the fish tank in its "comfortable" spot for three years, untouched, and threw *that* inside. Ed then reached for the unopened bar of Coast soap sitting next to the dog shampoo and chucked that inside the trash bag, too. He followed up with countless other artifacts that served solely as placeholders, keeping memories in real time—hats, T-shirts, old magazines, empty Gatorade bottles—and threw them all away. In that moment, Ed chose love, and Mayada, over the OCD that was always just one step behind him, trying to stand in his way. When the garbage bag was filled, he tied it in a knot, walked outside into the sunshine, and kicked the remnants of his old life to the curb.

Back inside, he grabbed another trash bag and headed toward his bed. Operating on pure adrenaline, he began rolling up the old foam egg crate and dirty linens, quickly pushing them deep into the green plastic. He pulled out old socks, T-shirts, and sweat-pants he had hoarded from the drawers of his bureau, previously thinking that they meant something in the scheme of time, and threw them into this second bag. In this moment of clarity, they were just clothes that, given continued power, could come between him and Mayada.

Ed continued this exorcism, and by the time he was done, there were ten contractor-sized trash bags sitting on the front curb of his house waiting to be hauled away.

Standing in his driveway, staring at the collective memories of the life that had held him hostage for so long, he remembers the joyful sound of birds chirping and feeling the sunshine of a brilliant summer's day against his back, and he suddenly felt what he could only describe as freedom.

That evening, when Mayada walked into the room, she was thrilled at the sight of the cleaned basement, but she claims she was not surprised. She says she *knew* that Ed could and would eventually do it—she just didn't know it would be this soon. Mayada saw his gesture of throwing out the *Running Man* laser disc as one of the greatest acts of love she could imagine. "Ed showed that he was ready to start making new memories," she says.

The insidiousness of OCD never goes away. It is a chameleon constantly changing colors and manifestations to find new ways to intrude in to the lives of its victims. The high of what he'd done eventually wore off, and even the extraordinary victory of the cleaning of the basement was fleeting, because Ed knew if he became complacent in his battle against OCD, he could easily lose the war, and everything he'd worked so hard to gain. But despite the continued struggle he faced, Ed was comforted by the fact that he knew Mayada's compassion would always break his fall.

**MAYADA AND ED WERE IN** love, and she spent every possible moment with him when she wasn't working. In addition to the typical challenges a new couple face, her integration into Ed's mental and physical life posed unique challenges. There was always the latent fear that she might do something that would trigger his anxiety and OCD. If, for example, Ed was sitting on the end of his bed and Mayada walked into the room in which the lights were off and flipped on the light as he started to stand up to greet her, it would "trap" him. Ed would have to stand perfectly still while he asked her to turn the light off. He would then reposition himself exactly as he was the second before she turned the light on. The repositioning would allow him an additional try to make the switch flip an even number of times before he could feel right—that his body was perfectly aligned. Mayada would stand perfectly still as he went through this process, devastated that she had done something to cause him anguish. When he was ready, he would ask her to flip the light switch. If he still didn't *feel* right, they would have to repeat the same procedure until everything was perfect.

Then there were the mealtime episodes. If, for example, Mayada sat down first and Ed sat down second, when they were finished, he would have to get up first to leave the table. If she got up first, he would feel trapped. If, however, Ed sat down first, and Mayada sat down afterward, there were no restrictions on her ability to get up and down throughout the course of the dinner because his OCD was in control of the space he occupied. Getting through the management of Ed's OCD together required the entire force of their love, attention, and communication. It was not something easily understood by others.

As far as Ed had come in the management of his OCD, the deep struggle for him—one that created what he describes as total "disgust" with himself and the situation—was fighting for a new life that included someone else. He hated putting Mayada through the paces of his OCD. He constantly asked himself, "Why can't I just be normal?"

But Mayada's frustration came for completely different reasons. She desperately wanted to make his life better, not add to his anxiety. "I came into *his* life, and I had to adjust to *him*, not the other way around," says Mayada. "He had just come out of being in a basement for over two years." Ed was acutely sensitive to the times she seemed to lack patience with his OCD, but in actuality, she says, she was thinking *I'm an idiot!*—guilt-stricken for having created a situation that triggered a ritual.

At the time Mayada met Ed, he'd only really been living in the outside world for a couple of months. He was like a baby learning to walk. "Ed was still trying to figure out how to be in the outside world without interfering with anyone's life," remembers Mayada. As he negotiated and modified his response to the demands of his OCD, Ed struggled to find ways to cope that would minimize its impact on his new life, and the lives of the people around him.

"Nighttime was always tough for Ed," says Mayada, "because he would filter the day out in his brain." There would be a long period of decompressing each night when Ed would zone out to rewind the mental videotape of the day's events. Internally, he would question all of his moves and then undo every little thing he had experienced during the day, by doing it over again. The rewinding, he feared, would be a chronic compulsion.

**WHEN MAYADA INTRODUCED ED TO** her family, she says their initial reaction was not warm. They didn't understand her accommodations—the calm voice, gentle touch, and reassurances she gave to Ed to calm his anxiety when he was in a new and stressful environment. She says there were members of her family who viewed her behavior as something *he* was controlling. The lack of understanding and acceptance from members of Mayada's family only served to raise Ed's anxiety, and the two would make a conscious decision to disengage from regular interactions as a defense mechanism to protect the life they were trying to build together.

Mayada worried about Ed, wondering if maybe everything was happening too fast for him. She says she would have waited months, and probably *years,* for him if he told her he needed more time to himself to manage his OCD. But she also knew that Ed was committed to their relationship and was doing everything he could to manage all the new changes in his life, and that she would not presume to make the decision of what he should do.

Working together to create a fresh environment downstairs, Ed and Mayada made a trip to Wal-Mart one night to buy cleaning products. Not surprisingly, whenever Ed went to a store—or *any* building for that matter—he had to walk *out* the same door he walked *in*. On this particular night, it was near closing, and while they were shopping, the manager locked every entrance but the one through which the remaining customers were allowed to exit. The lone unlocked door happened to be different from the one he had used to *enter* the store. Standing at the door through which he entered, in a panic, sweating, he wondered what he was going to do. He couldn't just walk through the door to the parking lot because that would be yet *another* door that he would have to walk through to complete the cycle. As his mind went on high-speed alert to calculate the different scenarios in which he might save himself, meet the demands of his OCD, and not cause an embarrassing scene in front of Mayada, he withdrew from talking at all, and "zoned" out. Mayada simply reached out and touched Ed's arm to let him know that everything was all right. This reassurance allowed his panic to subside long enough for him to walk over to the manager, explain his illness, and ask that he open up the other door so he could leave. The manager, very kindly, complied with Ed's request.

As Mayada and Ed left the store, his frustration with himself soared as he wondered, "Why can't I just walk in and out of doors like other people?" At that moment, he couldn't appreciate how far he'd come in being able to simply *come* to Wal-Mart and in continuing to be open about his illness. But Mayada knew, and she responded by reaching over, giving him a kiss, and telling Ed exactly how proud she was. "'You were willing to make the attempt when others might not,'" he remembers her saying. It was exactly what Ed needed to hear. She was, without doubt, the most influential person in his life since his mother.

**ED IS A HOPELESS ROMANTIC,** and Mayada was now the center of his world. He delighted in making plans for what he calls "an enchanted evening" to surprise her. It was just weeks since his surprise reintroduction to Michael Jenike, and Ed called him to share the news of the romantic carriage ride he had planned through historic Boston. Michael was surprised, but pleased that Ed was so happy, and he recalls having no concerns about the rapid progression of his relationship with Mayada.

In the warm night air of Boston, with roses in hand, Ed read Mayada a beautiful poem he'd written. Secretly, she was expecting a marriage proposal that night, and Ed suspected it. But he would wait just a little longer before giving her the romantic proposal he had already planned in the back of his mind.

The first week of August, Ed took Mayada to a footbridge overlooking Martha's Vineyard, near the place where they had shared their first date, and their first kiss, and bent down, feigning tying his shoelace. On bended knee, he looked up and said, "You give me all the reasons in the world to want to be whole again." Opening her hand, he placed something imaginary in her palm and said, "This is my heart, and it now belongs to you. Will you marry me?" Tears streamed down her cheeks; it was the moment she'd hoped would come since she first laid eyes on Ed walking down the sidewalk of the Landfall Restaurant. "Yes . . . yes . . . yes!" she cried.

The only people invited to the small private wedding ceremony were Mayada's mother, one of her sisters, and Ed's father. Their lives, their battle with OCD, and their future belonged to just them, and they needed protection from negative outside influence in the fragile early stages of their relationship. Together just three short months before their wedding, Ed says, "I wanted something just for me, maybe because this was something brand-new and refreshing." Ed wanted something simple to celebrate the landscape of his life, and a future that was wide open with possibilities. After spending a wonderful, weeklong honeymoon in New Hampshire, the newlyweds returned home to their first big challenge.

# CHAPTER 16

# In-Laws and OCD

⏪

THE FIRST YEAR OF MARRIAGE was a difficult one for Ed, Mayada, and her family as everyone tried to adjust to her new marriage, not to mention the extraordinary anxiety it caused Ed. "We didn't know anything about OCD, and we believed at the time Ed was isolating her and pulling her away from us," says an anonymous family member.

Although Mayada's loyalty remained with her new husband, she struggled to find ways to interact with her family so they could get to know the Ed that *she* knew; she truly believed they would come to love and appreciate him the way she did. But it seemed the more contact she and Ed had with her family— whether by phone or in person—the more tension it created at home between the couple. Following one heated discussion, Mayada asked Ed not to raise his voice.

"My OCD went haywire when Mayada asked me to talk softly," remembers Ed. He says it was the straw that broke the camel's back, and his OCD mind unloaded in the most extreme and illogical way it could. It demanded that he reverse the request she had made of him to erase the pain from what had been said. She would now have to speak even softer, and even more gently in order to accommodate his OCD, even though Ed knew, logically, that her request was reasonable. This was a clear expression of all the pent-up frustration and stress that was weighing on him. Mayada felt that if she and Ed were going to get through this difficult time together, and to protect him from further trauma, she would have to acquiesce and do OCD's bidding until it passed.

Remarkably, Mayada had managed to separate the OCD from Ed the person. She knew these demands were not part of the logical mind of her loving husband—she knew it came from an illogical place in his mind—and she felt the need to do whatever she felt would protect him from getting sicker. But to the uninformed, it *appeared* Ed was trying to control Mayada.

The one person in Mayada's family with whom Ed managed to form a relationship was, not surprisingly, her mother. Having lost his own mother at such an early age, this relationship was important to him, and he not only encouraged Mayada to stay close with her mother, even during these turbulent times with her family, he was insistent that after each visit, she not leave until she had given her mother a hug good-bye.

Growing up in Palestine with her father, Mayada says she was made to hug *everyone* good-bye as a sign of respect, whether she wanted to or not, but when she returned home to America to live with her mother, she dropped the tiresome habit. So when the family watched Ed insist Mayada do something that she would not ordinarily do, no matter how well intentioned, it *appeared* as though he was being controlling.

AS THE HAUNTING MONTHS OF November and December approached in that first year of Ed and Mayada's marriage, he began to think more persistently about the death of his mother, which caused even greater escalation of his anxiety and triggered the vicious cycle of OCD rituals he had seemingly gotten under control. He consequently became withdrawn and was unable to function the way he had in the spring when he and Mayada first met.

Mayada was deeply afraid for her husband that winter—worried that he would slip back into isolation and regress. She would come home directly after work and do everything she could to reassure him, and herself, that everything would be okay.

To complicate matters, she found out she was pregnant, and she didn't know how he was going to handle the news. That night, she walked into the living room, sat down on the sofa next to Ed, and put her hand on his knee just as she had the first time they met. She watched carefully for his reaction.

Ed's first reaction was one of pure joy, and he was immediately taken back to 1992, the same year he made eye contact with Mayada at TCBY, when he had a dream that one day he would have a daughter named Alexandria—and he was now certain that she was carrying a girl. They immediately embraced and kissed and basked in the wonderful news.

But Ed did sense Mayada's fear as she carefully monitored his reaction, and it was infectious. By the time the initial high wore off, and the obsessions kicked in, Ed began to panic. Was he going to be a good dad? *Could* he be a good dad? How was he going to handle a new baby coming into the new environment that he had created with Mayada? A baby would touch things, and move things, and he didn't know if his OCD could handle that. He wondered how life was going to change in other ways with a new baby in the house, and if they would be able to manage financially. More important, Ed had become dependent on the love and attention that Mayada showed him every day, and he wondered if that would change. He was sick, and needed her, and OCD was starting to play games in his head already; he knew it would only get worse. What if he wound up back in the basement, unable to function, with Mayada taking care of a child and a disabled husband and having to work full-time to support the family? It was the sadness he lived with in every moment of the day.

Ed expressed his concerns to Mayada, hoping she would address them calmly, with all of the same understanding he was used to. But Mayada's hormones were raging, and she was as frightened as Ed, in her *own* way, and things didn't go at all well.

"Sometimes I was a little too communicative," says Ed. He voiced his own fears about their future, and it only served to frighten Mayada even more. The thought of trying to manage their life, and his OCD, and her family with a baby became almost unbearable for her.

"I knew that Ed was already doing everything in his power to adjust to me being in his environment," says Mayada, "and now he would have to adjust all over again. I just didn't know how this would affect his health."

The rituals and the counting increased, tensions raised,

words flew between them. Mayada and Ed needed time to bond more slowly, instead of overnight, under these strained conditions and family kinds of pressure. The same went for her relationship with her family, who needed time to understand the pain of Ed's disorder.

"Everything was falling apart, and I just snapped," says Ed. "I felt I was getting hammered from the fights with my in-laws, and now the pregnancy." Soon Mayada moved back home with her mom to think things through.

IT HAD BEEN EXACTLY TWO years since Michael Jenike sat in Ed's living room feeling the weight of hopelessness in Ed's life, and he'd come so far, climbing mountains toward a life that was filled with love and hope for the future. But now, the opposing forces of OCD threatened to shut him down again. "Having fear of something can be paralyzing. It stops people from pursuing their dreams, and from functioning," says Ed. "And just like it stopped me from taking a shower, brushing my teeth, and living in the outside world, I was afraid of the changes that were about to take place."

Ed was poised to be stopped again. It was not a complete surprise to friends like Don Post, who were concerned about how quickly his life had changed.

"First I heard he'd gotten better," says Don, "then I heard he'd married, and now he was going to be a father. I was very concerned he'd have a major setback." As for Michael, who generally believes that when an OCD patient is ready to engage in ordinary activities, it's a very good sign, he saw that the pregnancy had caused extraordinary stress for Ed, and his concern grew, as well.

Ed had to find a way to use his technique of flipping the script on this, and fast, or he was going to lose everything he loved, and he was going to wind up in a place that he had worked so hard to escape. He truly believed that this pregnancy was their shared destiny, but the illogical mind of his OCD was doing everything in its power to tear it apart and take something away from him that was good. "Internally," he says, "it felt like *War of the Worlds* was playing in my head, because OCD (which Ed now consciously viewed as *his* enemy) viewed the baby as a threat, an interference trying to take over my life, and I was losing control."

Michael drove down to see Ed, and the two spent hours talking through his fears. During their discussion, Ed rationalized that the process of having a baby and being a father could only be accomplished successfully if he allowed himself to embrace the idea, just as he had embraced Mayada coming into his environment. If he could just wrap his head around the idea that he would be embracing a child in the same way, surely everything would be fine.

Ed managed to work through his fears, and Mayada was able to return home just a few days later to the husband she loved. The couple had to cocoon themselves emotionally for the next several months while Ed adjusted to the idea of his expanding family, and he was determined to give her the best first pregnancy experience possible.

"My wife was absolutely beautiful," gushes Ed. "When they say pregnant women glow, it's true. She looked like Lester the Light Bulb!"

As challenging as it was, Ed had once again triumphed in the face of adversity as he worked to put everything in perspective, just as he had done in the basement on the day he cleaned out his old life—only now it was a mantra that he played in his head repeatedly, "Mayada first, OCD second." Ed stepped up to the plate and began to dote on his wife as he had in the early days of their courtship. Mayada confirms that Ed successfully "made things so easy for me during the pregnancy. He was so wonderful and comforting."

From an outsider's perspective during this time, most people would not have guessed that Ed had OCD, because he worked so hard to suppress his illness and hide his rituals—for Mayada's sake. If she accidentally trapped him with the light, he suppressed the anxiety for as long as he could, then walked over to the light switch and flipped the toggle back and forth once she left the room. He did his touching and counting rituals privately, and though sometimes it was excruciating, he began waiting until she was out of the room before he walked backward up the steps to rewind his forward movements. He often sacrificed his own health because suppressing his rituals would increase his anxiety and result in even more ritualistic behavior. But he was determined to conceal his symptoms because he didn't want Mayada to have to deal with the "hiccups" caused by the disorder or be concerned that he was struggling. He wanted to make sure that she had a happy, healthy, worry-free pregnancy.

But the suppression of the OCD did cause the decompressing rituals to be more intense, and nighttime was a difficult time for him. There were times that he desperately needed their husband and wife time together at the end of the day so that he could find his comfort and words of reassurance, but finding that time was hard. Being pregnant, working full-time, and fielding phone calls from family members seeking their own reassurance that she was okay, Mayada, understandably, was so exhausted by the end of the night—when Ed needed her most—that all she could do was sleep.

Ed struggled as he wished there was a neutral third party that he could just vent to, but he refused to dishonor Mayada by talking about their business to family members and friends.

But Ed resolved to live for the joy he found in the little moments with Mayada during her pregnancy, and, of course, he tried to focus on all the positives about becoming a father. He remembers clearly the first visit to the midwife when they saw the baby through ultrasound. When Ed got excited and said, "Look Mayada, there she is," it was as if the baby knew that it was her daddy talking. She responded by turning her head directly toward him, and Ed responded back, crying, "Look, she's looking at me." This was his first communication with Alexandria. It was a moment—a very special moment.

They had all traveled a long, hard road to get to this point, and for all of the stress that had sometimes weakened his resolve to fight his OCD, this experience had just flipped that script, and he was empowered to continue his battle. More than ever, there was a something to fight for—to live a regular life with his family.

AT THREE O'CLOCK IN THE morning in October 2000, Mayada's labor put in motion the ticking of time that could no longer be controlled. There was no turning back or rewinding the moment that was about to bring the birth of his daughter. It wasn't easy, as Ed took his wife into the hospital, a place that triggers so many horrible memories from his past. Mayada remembers, "Ed put his sickness aside and focused on me to make sure everything was smooth and comfortable for me." Through it all, he never left her side, keeping his own fears in check long enough to cut the umbilical cord and hold his daughter for the first time. "I thought being married made me a man," says Ed, "but when I saw Alexandria, that's when I officially became a man."

The birth of Alexandria Irene Zine was a joyous occasion, marred by only a few rituals when Ed had to negotiate different elevators to get up and down the hospital floors and had to do some retracing and repetitions. And since new mothers have to leave from a different side of the hospital, Ed found himself having to go back and reroute himself through all the hospital entrances and exits before he could drive away with his wife and baby girl.

But once Alexandria was home, Ed became as doting a father as he was a husband. In fact, at night, previously the most trying time of the day for Ed, he actually looked forward to taking turns to feed and burp the baby.

When Mayada's mother once asked her if she was concerned about Alexandria picking up the habit of Ed's rituals, she responded by saying, "We may live with OCD, but our lives are more normal than most people, because as a person, Ed is a million times better than most people."

# CHAPTER 17

# A Choice of Dreams

⏮

ED WAS CONSUMED WITH THE responsibilities and joy of fatherhood. His life had come full circle, and when he held Alexandria in his arms, he knew what it meant to be a true hero.

As a new father, protecting Alexandria meant not allowing the demands of his OCD to affect her and adversely impact her world. Whether it was feeding her, burping her, or changing her diaper, he refused to indulge in his rituals. "OCD became like a switch," he says. "When I was with my daughter, I turned it off—it was instinctive—I didn't want even a hint of my OCD being around her, because she was just beginning her life."

Michael Jenike's advice to parents with OCD is that they should "protect their children from overt rituals." Children do learn through observation, and he says if they have a genetic tendency toward OCD, this could bring it out.

This is, of course, easier said than done. Ed's ability to compartmentalize his OCD and turn it off, or keep it at bay when he was with Alexandria—and Isabella, who was born in January 2005—did not mean that it had gone away. But, once again, he was finding ways to negotiate and manage its impact on his life. The need to stop the progression of time went away because now, perhaps, rather than having a *perceived* responsibility for the life of a parent, or sibling, he had the very *real* responsibility for the life of his child, and he was completely invested in seeing her grow up happy and healthy. "Being a parent gave me more balance," says Ed. "I now had a center of gravity—it assisted me in giving me strength where my weaknesses were."

Mayada and Alexandria gave Ed a purpose, and vision for the future, and he had some very practical decisions to make in his new role as patriarch of his growing family about how he was going to support them and build the kind of life he wanted for them.

ED'S PASSION IS HIS ART, and he still harbored the dream of becoming an animation artist. The fact that OCD had never affected Ed's ability to draw is inexplicable. Even in his deepest, darkest days, he was never burdened by the rituals that invaded every other area of his life . . . he never felt compelled to rewind and repeat his pencil strokes. Art was his freedom of expression, and it gave him a landing place for his emotions, dreams, and frustrations. He began to think that going back to school to pursue a career in art was the answer.

In the spring of 2000, with Mayada's full support, Ed began researching schools and putting together a portfolio of work for submission. When he finally decided to apply to the School Museum of Fine Art (SMFA) in Boston, neither he nor Mayada had any idea how they would manage such a dream with a new baby on the way if it were to become a reality, but they were both ready to try.

After submitting his application, Ed spoke with the director of admissions for SMFA and told her about his personal battle with OCD. Soon, with Ed's permission, she was on the phone with Michael Jenike to get a reference. Interestingly, Michael had treated a couple of patients at the OCD Institute who were also students at SMFA, and he knew that in spite of their OCD, they were doing quite well in school. He had seen Ed's artwork—in fact, Ed had done a couple of drawings for Michael and had given them to him as a gift—and he not only believed in Ed's talent, he believed in his resolve.

In the late summer of 2000, on the drive from Cape Cod to Boston, with Mayada by his side, Ed held in his hand a letter of acceptance to the School Museum of Fine Arts. During his visit to the campus to meet the director of admissions to discuss the financial commitment that would be required should he choose to attend, Ed was filled with mixed emotions. As he walked around campus, holding Mayada's hand, he knew that this place held every possibility for him to realistically pursue his art and live his dream.

But what about his other dream? When Mayada became pregnant, Ed started picking up jobs in construction, and he was making good money now. He had a chance to buy his father's house and actually own a piece of the American dream for his family. He was nervous about taking out a school loan, moving to Boston, renting a place, and giving up work.

The decision was completely his. Ed knew he had Mayada's full support either way—but while the first questions on his mind concerned the right thing to do for his *family* and his ability to support them while attending school (could he manage working construction jobs on the Cape while attending school in Boston?), he also wondered how many times he would have an opportunity like this.

Throughout his bout with OCD, Ed frequently employed the visual of the scales of justice whenever he was torn by a diffi-cult decision, and in the early days of his retreat from the base-ment, he envisioned two simple, however significant, influences in his life, which he placed on either side of the scale: Mayada and OCD—and he always chose Mayada. But now there were multiple sides of the equations of his life to consider . . . Mayada, Alexandria, OCD, work, and art school. Back home, as Ed sat alone at the table staring at the envelope with the SMFA logo that held his acceptance letter, he faced the crushing weight of having to make a choice between two dreams.

DURING MAYADA'S PREGNANCY, WHEN ED first decided to try and go back to the world of construction, he wondered how he would negotiate the demands of his disorder. He knew he couldn't escape his rituals completely, and he wondered how he would be accepted by the guys on the job when they found out about his OCD.

Phil Miller, his friend from the gym who owned a construction company and one of the few people to support Ed in his Clemson endeavor years before, had suffered his own tragedy as a young man. After graduating from Georgetown University, he was involved in a terrible accident and lost one of his legs, so he understood what it was like to get knocked on your ass at a time when you're just starting to try to make your dreams a reality. Although he didn't know how well Ed would function on the job, Phil sure didn't mind giving a guy like him a chance, as he recalled Ed's resolve to attend Clemson and the physical results of that early training. Ed, Phil knew, was determined.

So Phil took Ed under his wing and allowed him to train himself on the Bobcat. Within weeks, he'd not only mastered it, but he was working it with such remarkable precision it was as if he'd been doing it all his life. At first, there was a little resentment among the other guys who thought Ed was getting special attention, afraid that he was being groomed to replace them. But as they got to know Ed and he openly shared the details of his OCD, they actually had compassion and even admiration for him, and he soon become one of the guys.

But being "one of the guys" meant, OCD or no OCD, you were going to get your chops busted on a regular basis. Billy Valadao, an electrician who worked with Ed, remembers, one time, standing inside a construction site with the other guys watching Ed drive by, and they all stood there counting the seconds before he had to drive backward past the window again. But Billy says that though there may have been a few complaints about all the extra gas Ed used to satisfy his rituals, everyone mostly just joked about them good-heartedly, and Ed took it all in stride.

After a while, Ed's OCD was just something everyone accepted and lived with. Billy would often pick Ed up for work so he could leave the car with Mayada, and he would always care-fully plan out the route to their construction site the night before so that they could avoid rotaries and left-hand turns. When they were working at an estate site with separate entrances to enter and exit, Billy would make a point to drive *into* the site the wrong way in the morning (that is, through the exit), so when they left in the afternoon, they could simply drive out the right way, and Ed would be okay.

When he prepared the work schedule every day, Phil typically made a point to never schedule Ed on a job on Martha's Vineyard. He knew that Ed couldn't go work in a place where they had to take a ferry or travel roads that went only one way around an island that prevented him from reversing the drive. But one Sat-urday morning, he forgot.

**IT WAS 5:30 IN THE** morning when Ed pulled up in front of Phil's house in the company dump truck. "So where are we headed?" asked Ed. Phil told Ed that they were going to the Vineyard.

Ed's panic was instant. Consumed by fear, his heart started racing, adrenaline rushed through his body, and he started freak-ing out right in front of Phil. He couldn't do it, he told Phil—no way—it wasn't going to happen. There was no way he could drive the dump truck to Martha's Vineyard. It was the last thing in the world he wanted to do to the guy who'd done so much to help him learn the business and get back on his feet—but he couldn't comply. His OCD wouldn't let him.

Phil didn't know what to do. He hated seeing Ed like this, but he had a business to run, and a job to do. There were guys waiting on the island, counting on the two of them to get over there with this equipment. Phil stood firm. "We're all ready to go, Eddie," he said. "We gotta go, so we're going."

Ed's head was exploding—everything felt wrong—screeching nails in his head—everything was spinning around—he felt nauseous and scared. What would happen to Mayada and Alexandria? Ed was so upset that he could barely hear what Phil was saying. "It's too late, Eddie; I have commitments, we've got to go." Ed was trying so hard to scan his mind for those movies, those peaceful moments, the happier memories that would help ease his anxiety.

Finally, he calmed down enough to say, "Okay, can I ask you a favor?" At this point, Phil was pissed off—everyone else was already at the job—what was he going to do? Miss a whole day's work because Ed couldn't drive to Martha's Vineyard?

"What?" he asked, gruffly.

"Will you hold my hand?" Ed asked meekly.

Phil looked at Ed and took a deep breath. The terror in Ed's face was real—all logic had escaped him—and he was in the panicked grip of OCD. Phil realized that holding Ed's hand, no matter how uncomfortable an idea it might have been for both men, was a small thing to ask. Besides, what choice did Phil have?

"Sure, buddy," Phil said in a calmer voice. "I'll hold your hand."

"Can you imagine?" remembers Phil, smiling. "Two big construction guys in this big dump truck hauling a friggin' Bobcat, driving down the road and holding hands?"

Asking for Phil's hand wasn't an easy choice for Ed to make, but his resolve was strong, and he did what he had to do because he had a family counting on him at home.

# CHAPTER 18

# Building Dreams into Reality

◀◀

E**D HAD A CHOICE BETWEEN** two dreams—pursuing his art, which meant putting his family's comfort and financial security on hold, or staying the course and continuing to work in construction so he could buy the home that he wanted for his wife and child. In the end, memories of those summer days of his childhood playing in the backyard of the home where his father worked so hard to provide for his family, along with the carefree moments by his mother's side, helped to inform his choice. Life had come full circle—it was his turn to put his family first.

BY THE TIME ED WALKED into the office of home builder Brian Dacey in the spring of 2007, he was the father of two little girls, Alexandria Irene and Isabella Grace. The homes Brian was selling were way out of Ed's price range, but it was the perfect location to raise a family, so he thought he'd just go in and have a look— perhaps he could talk with Brian about buying a plot of land and building *his own* house. Not that he'd ever built a house before, or even been a general contractor, but he had a vision of what he wanted, and he'd been watching Phil build houses for years, so Ed was pretty sure he could do it if he set his mind to it. And why not? How many people would have been able to overcome the obstacles he'd already overcome?

Brian remembers that day. "Ed was a good-looking kid," he says, "and he was so sincere about trying to get his family into a home. I had to at least take the time to listen to what he had to say." Ed sat with Brian and poured his heart out. He told him about his OCD, being stuck in the basement and working his way out, and of course about Mayada and the girls.

Making a deal like this was important to Ed, not because he needed to live in a fancy, upscale home, but because he knew that if he could work it out to buy the land, he could build the house for cost and wind up with double the amount of home equity. This meant that if he ever got sick again and became unable to work—not something he liked to think about, but something for which he wanted to be prepared—Mayada and the girls would have the security they needed.

Brian was moved by Ed's story, but the problem was that he was a general contractor himself—he built estate neighborhoods and *never* split up plots of land and sold them to outside contractors. Ed managed to convince him that he was capable of building his own house to the same specs and with the same quality of construction that would match the rest of the homes in the neighborhood. And after three more meetings, where Ed showed up with everything he'd been asked to provide, Brian Dacey, against the presumably *better* judgment of his advisers, sold Ed the piece of land he wanted. Brian gave Ed an opportunity for which he says he is "eternally grateful."

Things like this didn't happen with upscale builders like Brian—everyone, including veterans of construction like Phil and Ed's dad, were in awe of what Ed managed to accomplish in getting him to sell a parcel of premium land on the Cape. Not surprisingly, Ed says there were friends and family members all around who openly wondered how he planned to general contract a house when he'd never done it before. But Ed was used to naysayers, and it didn't matter to him—he knew what he was capable of, and his job was to be the hero for his little girls. Even if OCD kicked his ass, he was determined to stay strong and make this home happen for them.

**DURING THE PLANNING AND BUILDING** stages of their new home, the demands on Ed's time and attention grew exponentially, and he struggled to juggle everything coming at him. Mayada worried that it was too much. "If you give me the choice of having a large luxury home and having Ed in good health, I choose my husband," she says. But she believes that Ed is still his own best guide in navigating the conflicts of his mind and fighting back his OCD. She will not tell him what to do.

As the pressure mounted, Ed constantly worked through the

maze of anxiety by honing his mental strategies and visualization skills. He says that he began to project images in his mind of all the potential negative scenarios related to any decision he had to make, and, in an instant, he could see every angle and process every potential outcome, to try and outwit his OCD. Conversations became particularly trying during this stressful time, but he continuously searched for ways to counteract the negative thoughts.

While talking with Mayada, for example, Ed says his brain will scan for visuals of acceptable words to use so he doesn't offend or upset her in any way, like Arnold Schwarzenegger in *Terminator*. Using his peripheral vision, he says, he looks up toward the outside of his left eye and sees a huge video screen in his mind that displays a list of words. If he looks to the outside of his right eye, the screen contains a list of appropriate responding actions he can take. Compartmentalizing the two, he scans for compatible scenarios that could play out in the most appeasing and positive way possible to accommodate his OCD and the person to whom he is speaking. Certain blocks pop up, indicating that a word is suitable, or signaling other potential problems with the combination of words and actions. As he structures his sentences making sure to use each word twice, and repeating them back and forth in his thoughts, he is responding internally to each word, *yes, no, yes, yes, no, no,* while at the same time trying to carry on a conversation, recording what is being said so he can rewind it later during his decompression period before he goes to bed.

Sometimes, the conscious Ed says yes to a word that pops up, but his OCD says, "No!" When the no's happen, OCD punishes Ed by making him find multiple acceptable words. "Go back, look again, yes, yes, yes, yes, NO!" If Ed's thoughts go into overload, he begins to internalize his thoughts and goes silent. Ed suspects the person to whom he is speaking will wonder why he stopped talking, and whether the silence is a signal that he is disinterested or just downright rude. But in this moment of limbo, Ed has a voice screaming in his head, "I CAN'T TALK, I CAN'T SPEAK . . . I'M DEALING WITH MY SICKNESS RIGHT NOW . . . SORRY!" At the same time, there is more punishment, and Ed must still repeat sentences backward, countless numbers of times: "!YRROS . . . WON THGIR SSENKCIS YM HTIW GNILAED M'I . . . KAEPS T'NAC I ,KLAT T'NAC I" But Ed cannot physically speak to tell the person that he is actually in the moment doing his reversing protocol in his head.

Anxieties multiply simultaneously, Ed says, as he scans the screen above his right eye for actions that may be associated with the revolving lists of words on the left screen, or simply rewinding events that occurred earlier in the day. Did he walk the same pattern through the door of the building, and then reverse it when he came out? Rewind. When his workout routine at the gym was interrupted by a conversation with friends, did he end his repetitions on an even number? Rewind. Ed struggles not to let his guard down, as he tries to capture every one of his rewinding routines, while still engaging in the real world and having real conversations. If he gets behind, he will get overwhelmed with trying to catch up, and then get locked down. He has to make peace with his actions, negotiating compromises and shortcuts wherever possible, but he can't just forget about them.

Ed says there are other tricks that he uses to keep his mind from imploding when he is overwhelmed. He imagines a piece of paper in his head, and on it is written all of his repetitious cycling thoughts and responsibilities. He mentally reviews the list and then crumples it up in his hand and throws it away, telling himself that all that stuff is gone and doesn't mean a thing. Whatever was weighing him down no longer exists. The audio track in his head telling him that everything will work itself out calms him, as he makes the continual choice not to slide into negative thinking, choosing to be happy, and attend to the problems one at a time.

There were many times throughout the course of building their new home that Ed wasn't sure even his most incredible mental strategies could save him from relapse. But almost every day that he was out working the land and building the house, his father was there by his side, giving him the benefit of his experience as a master builder. In the most profound compliment he can give, Bob says, "My son doesn't back away from nothing. He's brilliant."

IN DECEMBER OF 2007, ED, Mayada, and their two daughters moved into their brand-new home on Cape Cod. Started with a vision and realized with determination, this house Ed created with his own two hands is the culmination of a triumph of spirit.

Here, Ed, Mayada, and his girls have begun their new life. Ed still counts and checks, but he rarely gets stuck anymore. In his new home, he keeps things in an order that makes sense to him, but personal concern for their safety notwithstanding, he doesn't limit his children when they play. He no longer hoards items from his past to hold a place in time. At times, when Ed's anxiety rises and he finds himself having to walk backward, he acquiesces to the compulsion but carefully conceals it from his daughters. When he plays with them, he will pick them up, give them a hug and a kiss, turn around, and put them back down—that way he has unbound himself, addressed his OCD, and they're none the wiser.

When Ed walks up the basement steps of their new home, the ones that *he* built, he can walk straight into the sunshine where his daughters play in their new backyard, and he is at home. With Mayada by his side, he is living the heroic life he chose for himself, and a life of importance that his mother had predicted.

# CHAPTER 19

# Ed's Moment of Triumph

◀◀

AROUND 2003, MICHAEL ASKED ED if he would speak to a group of doctors on Cape Cod about his experience with obsessive-compulsive disorder, though he still didn't quite understand how Ed had managed to get unstuck from the basement. There was still an inexplicable disconnect in the way the two communicated about their shared experience. Michael was not able to dissect the scientific hows and whys of what had happened because Ed, as brilliant as he is, had always focused on the *emotional and intellectual* aspects of his miraculous recovery rather than the *clinical*.

In spite of the fact that Michael didn't fully understand the transformation, the message Michael wanted so desperately to send that day was that even the most severe OCD patients are capable of getting better and must not be ignored. The audience comprised a group of medical providers from all over the world whom, he says, might not normally put much effort into treating severe OCD patients, and they *certainly* weren't in the habit of going to a patient's home or giving their time gratis if they couldn't bill an insurance company for the visit.

Michael knew that if the most severe cases of OCD stand any chance at all, more doctors are going to have to be inspired to break out of the traditional medical model that currently exists, be willing to break the rules, and go to the home of a patient who is suffering. During his talks, he implores his fellow caregivers to *give* of their time and help take care of these underserved patients. "Everyone," he says, "can afford to do a little bit of charity."

Whether Michael understood it scientifically or not, Ed had a great story to tell. He had physically transformed from a frail, sick patient into a handsome, physically fit young man; he was functioning in the real world; and he had a beautiful wife and daughter (this was still two years before the birth of Isabella). He was a wonderful example of someone who had been severely, and hopelessly ill, and had managed to make his way into not only a productive life, but also one that even a healthy person could be proud of. As he introduced Ed to the crowd of about sixty health-care professionals, mostly physicians, Michael figured he would have to prompt Ed to talk about some of the more difficult details of his struggle, but he was shocked when Ed voluntarily stood up and asked Michael to sit down.

When Ed looked around the room, it was as if he had prepared all his life for this important moment. He wasn't afraid, he was ready. For the next hour, the room was in absolute silence as Ed shared the story of his deeply isolated life among the treasures of his past, and how he believed he was able to stop the progression of time and death. He recounted the ways in which Michael's honor and integrity broke through a mental and emotional wall, allowing him to begin reworking the way his obsessive thoughts could be controlled and managed. He explained the negotiations he did in his mind to combat the self-doubt and intrusive thoughts. He made the audience in front of him laugh and cry. Ed broke his OCD down with such precision that, afterward, he was told by a participant that "it was like someone had put a doctor inside of you to explain it; well done."

When he came to the end of his story, thunderous applause rang through the room and he received a standing ovation, and Michael watched in amazement, thinking over their history, incredulous that Ed had achieved such an overwhelming victory, and that the time lines of their lives had crossed in such an inexplicable way.

In this astounding moment, Ed knew he had achieved the one great thing his mother always believed he was destined to do.

◀◀

*In many ways, OCD is about integrity—you always have to do everything the right way, by the rules. There are a lot of rules.*

*One of the things I feel about OCD is that it analyzes too much. It picks apart every aspect of every conversation. It gets a foothold on you while you are consumed by everything else. It worries too much about the things we've done, are doing, or are going to do, all at the same time. While you're thinking you can take on the whole world all at the same time, you can't because OCD is tearing you down, filling you with self-doubt, making you unable to take just one step forward. We lock down and freeze.*

*If we could just simply drop all the worry, and do one thing at a time, we could start building successes on top of one another, but* we can't. All we can think about is what we can't do, and what we should be accomplishing—we can't process the whole load—and that's where we freeze. OCD is like a series of hiccups . . . it makes us think we can do more than we can, but then tells us, "No, I don't think you can." When we take one step back, and falter, we're filled with guilt and anxiety. Then, we get depressed.

The mind is a fickle and funny thing, a computer that processes people's lives, the way they live, the way they die, good times, and bad times. I believe that our brain is almost conducive for OCD to happen. Just like we all have a hero living inside of us, a stranger to our everyday persona—that person who would throw himself in front of a bus to protect a child—it's instinctive. I think that OCD can live inside of us and it's the flip side of the persona that shows up when someone is sick with this disorder—a stranger to our everyday persona—who appears selfish and demanding. What is the "born on" date of OCD? Is it trauma and stress? The rules and regulations are not set. We only learn about OCD and how to manage it as we go along, because it is different for everybody. But disabled means un-able, and unable is not a permanent.

OCD is just a word, but when it sucks the life out of my life, it also sucks the life out of my loved ones' lives. It is ruthless in its attack. When it hits you, it will not stop. We know that we are acting crazy, but we also know that we are not crazy. And while the outside world tries to take care of us, and reassure us, OCD spits in their faces, and tries to change, dictate, and control the ones who bring us love and reassurance.

Don Post once told me that an astronomer can look at the moon all day long and never know what it's like to walk in the shoes of an astronaut. The same goes for OCD—you can talk about it all day long, but until you've lived it you will never know the agony and the pain.

I owe so much to my wife, and her perspective is invaluable to me.

*Mayada's perspective:*

*It is the greatest honor for a person who lives with OCD to allow you into their delicate balance of life. It is only when they let go of their fears, and embrace the relationship, that true healing begins for them to move forward in life.*

◀◀

I HAVE SPENT NEARLY TWO years dissecting the relationship that formed between the two extraordinary men I have written about in this book as I assessed the remarkable transformation of Ed Zine.

In sharing this story with family and friends, the question everyone asks is, "What *exactly* did Michael do to make Ed better?"

The answer is as simple as it is complicated.

First, Ed is not cured of OCD. He has made the transformation from a helpless, hopeless victim of this insufferable disorder to survivor. He is a man who fights every minute of every day to manage the impact of OCD so he can live his best life with his family. And as shocking as it may sound, Michael did not make Ed better—Ed fought the fight and made himself better.

*But* if Michael had not been willing to make that house call— if he had not been willing to bring the full force of his humanity, understanding, and compassion to bear; if he had not been willing to bring to Ed the best therapy medicine had to offer, and exhaust every possible avenue to *try* and make him better—Ed may never have reached that critical turning point where *he* was willing to fight to make himself better.

And, at the end of the day, what worked for Ed was a process rooted in the fundamentals of traditional cognitive behavioral therapy (CBT) and exposure and response prevention (ERP) therapy. Wittingly—or unwittingly—the treatment that Ed designed and customized to meet his own needs was the same therapy Michael would have practiced with him had he been able to go to the OCD Institute.

A man whom I will cherish for the rest of my days once told me, "Evil triumphs when good men do nothing." In that statement, as unscientific as it may be, lies the answer. Michael came home a hero from a war and did something that led him on a journey over time to the house on Cape Cod and allowed Ed to triumph.

I have had the extraordinary honor of sharing the company of these two heroes for the past two years as they have graciously opened up their families, and the most painful experiences of their lives, to me. From a day of yachting on the rough waters off the Atlantic coast with Michael and Una, to driving around the Cape with Ed and Mayada to see the first breaking of ground at the site of their new home, it has been a deeply personal experience.

The OCD experience is also a deeply personal experience for me and my family.

My son, Patrick, was seventeen years old when he was first diagnosed with OCD. Coincidentally, seventeen years is the same amount of time it takes for the average sufferer to get a correct diagnosis. Patrick suffers from "just right" OCD and obsessive worry. He is a perfectionist for whom anything less is, in his own words, "like nails being driven into my brain." And even though he demonstrated signs of OCD from a very young age, I didn't know his symptoms had a name.

Even as I wrote this book, I found myself hanging up the phone with Ed to take an international call from Patrick who was studying in Italy and struggling with OCD so profound that he was unable to move from one line of text to the next for a full hour, unsure if he'd read it perfectly.

Writing this book made me think of the years of endless sleepless nights as my son lay awake until two, three, and four o'clock every morning replaying the day's events in his mind, and obsessively worrying about what *might* happen at school the next day. Sunday nights were excruciating as he worried not just about the next day, but about the *whole* week ahead. He tried so hard not to come in and wake me up, but it didn't matter, I lay down the hall listening to him toss and turn, get up and down out of bed, and turn on the light to read so he could distract himself from worry.

Eventually, he would knock on my door, and apologize for the reassurances that he so desperately wanted—the voice that he needed to hear say, "it's okay"—over, and over, and over again. For years, we both operated on less than four to five hours of sleep a night—until Friday came. He didn't worry about Saturdays so much, and he'd sleep—and I would sleep—as long as we could. I was often criticized for being a mother who allowed her son to "sleep all day long." But we were simply exhausted.

Friends and family whose own children simply dropped into bed and fell asleep—something for which I constantly prayed—would offer suggestions that I should punish Pat, ignore him, or lock him in his room and refuse to let him get up or read. Believe me, I tried a few times, but his anxiety level would skyrocket, and he wouldn't sleep at all. So I compromised and accommodated because he desperately needed to get *some* sleep in order to make it through the next day and stay healthy.

Had I only known it was OCD, and that the best treatment is *not* to accommodate, and that exposure and prevention therapy would eventually quell the obsessive and compulsive behaviors, I would have tried *not* to accommodate so much. But even then, for a family member witnessing such suffering, and he did suffer, giving reassurance is not easy to resist.

As a child, Patrick was rarely comfortable in his clothes—he would find one outfit that felt okay, and he wanted to wear it every day. When I insisted that he change, my otherwise gentle and obedient child would suddenly become hysterical and throw a fit. He told me, even then, that his clothes didn't *feel* right, but that didn't make sense to me after trying everything to make sure they were comfortable. I would buy soft clothes—sweatpants—and change detergents thinking maybe he was allergic. I spoke to his pediatrician, his grandmother, anyone who might help me figure out why this was such an issue—but no one had an answer.

Finally, I resorted to buying five outfits exactly the same, and I washed them the exact same numbers of time to try and trick him—but even that didn't work. He knew the difference.

When I demanded that he put on fresh clothes, he would kick and scream and pull his belt so tight around his waist that I actually thought he might damage his kidneys. I would punish him with time-outs for what I thought was bad behavior. But Patrick recently explained that tightening his belt was a distraction from the "pain" of his pants not *feeling* just right; that *feeling* was absolute torture for him.

When I spoke to his pediatrician about Pat's sleepless nights, he was simply, generically, labeled a "worrier." This label actually took a dangerous turn when symptoms of a serious, but intermittent, heart issue were ignored by his pediatrician who thought his light-headedness and "racing heart" was caused by worry.

It was by chance, or fate, that I met Michael Jenike on a consulting project and began to get a peripheral understanding of OCD. The more I learned, the more I wanted to learn because it all sounded much too familiar. Ultimately, he began seeing Patrick as a patient, and Pat was finally given a diagnosis, and relief knowing there was a rhyme and reason to his illogical behavior. Having the behavioral tools to help him manage his OCD and get through the stressful times has made all the difference.

I know, without a doubt, that the quality of Patrick's life would have been significantly greater had we only known. Today, he is a successful college senior and headed to law school after Boston College, and he no longer suffers in silence as countless millions of other male, female, and child sufferers do.

"I didn't know." These are the words I use to describe my personal experience as a mother of a child with OCD, and they are the same exact words Bob Zine repeated to me during his first emotional interview about his son.

For parents and family members reading this story—it doesn't have to be that way. I encourage you to go to: www.ocfoundation. org to find out more.